Let's go a walk

Rebuilding body, mind and spirit after a stroke

THOMAS GRAHAM

with illustrations by
Slobodanka Graham

© 2025 Thomas Graham
Published by BG Publishers
www.bgpublishers.com.au

All rights reserved.

Text and cover design by Dhiraj Navlakhe
Digital edition by SunTecIndia
Printed by IngramSpark

First edition 2025

ISBN (print) 9781763772120
ISBN (digital) 9781763772137

*Stroke Survivors . . .
believe in your recovery
practice movement, daily
be patient and
kind to yourself*

CONTENTS

Medical emergency

Life turned upside down	10
Introduction	15

Part one
Day one to twenty-two

Day one	21
Day two	22
Day three	24
Day four	26
Day five	28
Day six	29
Day seven	30
Day eight	31
Day nine	32
Day ten	34
Day eleven	36
Day twelve	37
Day fourteen	39
Day fifteen	40
Day twenty	42
Day twenty-two	43

Part two
Post-stroke recovery: physical

Day fifteen	
An arm and a leg	47
Day twenty-three	
The power to heal	52

Day forty-three
  Walking backwards into the future   76
Day fifty-five
  Letter in response to Bobby's
  friend, a long term yoga teacher   84
Day sixty-three
  Letter in response to a
  South African friend   88
Day sixty-six
  'Brindy' rehab   92
Day eighty-five
  Three Months   105
Day one hundred and eighty-five
  Entering the age of senescence   108

Part three
Ongoing recovery: body, mind and spirit

Day two hundred and seventy-three
  Sweet, Green Sit Spot   121
Day two hundred and eighty-eight
  Bare Feet   124
Day two hundred and eighty-nine
  Agitation   125
Day two hundred and ninety-two
  Fireside Friendships   126
Day two hundred and ninety-four
  Wagga on my mind   128
Day two hundred and ninety-five
  Befriending an Oak   130
Day two hundred and ninety-six
  Anticipation   132
Day three hundred and four
  Leap Year   135

Day three hundred and eighteen Changing Seasons	137
Day three hundred and twenty-seven Double Delight	139
Day three hundred and twenty-seven Lunar Readings	142
Day three hundred and thirty-four Misty Dawn	144
Day three hundred and forty-eight First Mist	146
First Anniversary of Stroke Becoming One	148
Day three hundred and sixty-nine Statin Intolerance	150
Day three hundred and eighty-five First Frost	152
Day three hundred and eighty-seven Anniversary Moon	154
Day three hundred and ninety-six Nature's Maxim	156
Day three hundred and ninety-seven Hall to Home	157
Day four hundred and two Winter Solstice	160
One year, two months Pathways to Physical Restoration	162
Day four hundred and thirty-five Aqua Refresh	179
Day four hundred and thirty-seven Unmasked	181
Day four hundred and forty Westbourne Woods	183

Day four hundred and forty-six	
Haiku Moment	185
Day four hundred and forty-eight	
Every circle has a centre	186
Day four hundred and fifty-one	
West Wind	188
One year, three months	
Remembering Bojangles	189
One year, four months	
Refreshed and energised by nature	194
Day . . .	
The future	211
Thank you	215
Glossary	219
Resources cited and courses completed	221
Medical alert!	223

Medical emergency

Life turned upside down

Tuesday, 2 May 2023
Osprey Road, Harrison, ACT

A mid-morning drive
as Mr Petman
to Benny, feline friend
devoted family pet.

I unload tools from ute
to begin work
reconnecting cat tunnel
to new double-glazed window
with cat door.

An hour passes before
an unfamiliar sensation arises
light headedness, faint dizziness
internal unease, puzzlement.

I return to my ute
limbs laboured, climbing into cab
pour a cup of tea
sipping the Earl Grey
I sense not being right.

Speaking out loud to myself
I hear my words, they're slurred
Confused, I phone Bobby
she hears my vocal discord
makes the connection: stroke
'I'll call an ambulance'
'No! You pick me up'.

We arrive at Calvary Hospital
I remain in car, outside of Emergency
"I think my husband has had a stroke!"
The triage nurse opens the car door
looks at me, calls it.
Immediately, a medical team responds.

Placed in a wheelchair, I'm taken inside
stripped of sweat-laden clothes
my steel-capped boots removed
an intravenous drip inserted into my arm.

A doctor questions Bobby
'What happened, when, where?'
I'm asked to lift my arms, my legs
to follow the doctor's moving finger with my eyes
left to right, right to left
Do I know what day it is, where I am?

Sent for a scan, the result inconclusive
the neurologist is called
She makes the decision, no delay
administer the clot-buster medication.

In the aftermath, I'm wheeled to the lift
taken up to Level 5B
admitted into acute care
the Stroke Unit, Bed 34.

My (our) life is shaken
turned upside down
No ordinary day
a long night awaits
tomorrow uncertain.

| 2 MAY
| TUESDAY

STR

OUR WORLD SHIFTED FOREVER WHEN THOMAS HAD A STROKE. IT WAS LIKE A DEVASTATING **EARTHQUAKE** OF HIS BODY AND OUR SOULS.

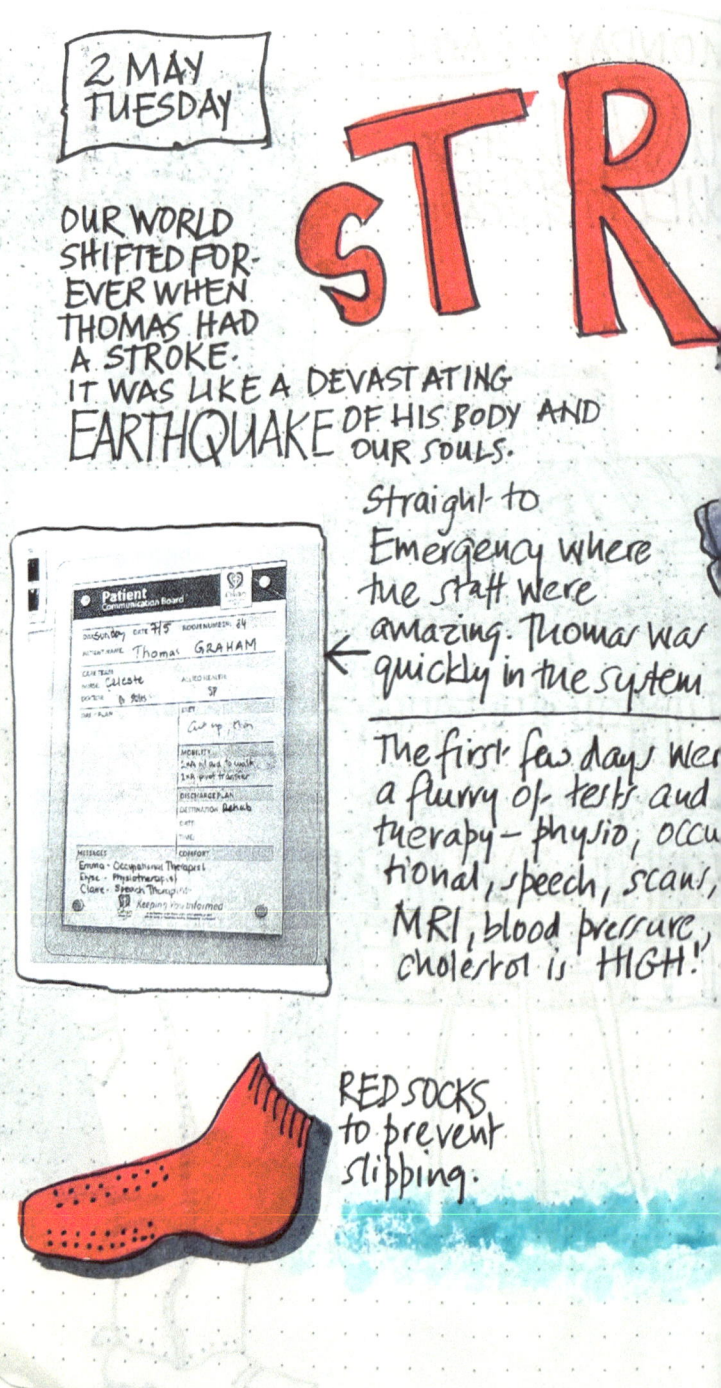

Straight to Emergency where the staff were amazing. Thomas was quickly in the system.

The first few days were a flurry of tests and therapy — physio, occupational, speech, scans, MRI, blood pressure, cholesterol is HIGH!

RED SOCKS to prevent slipping.

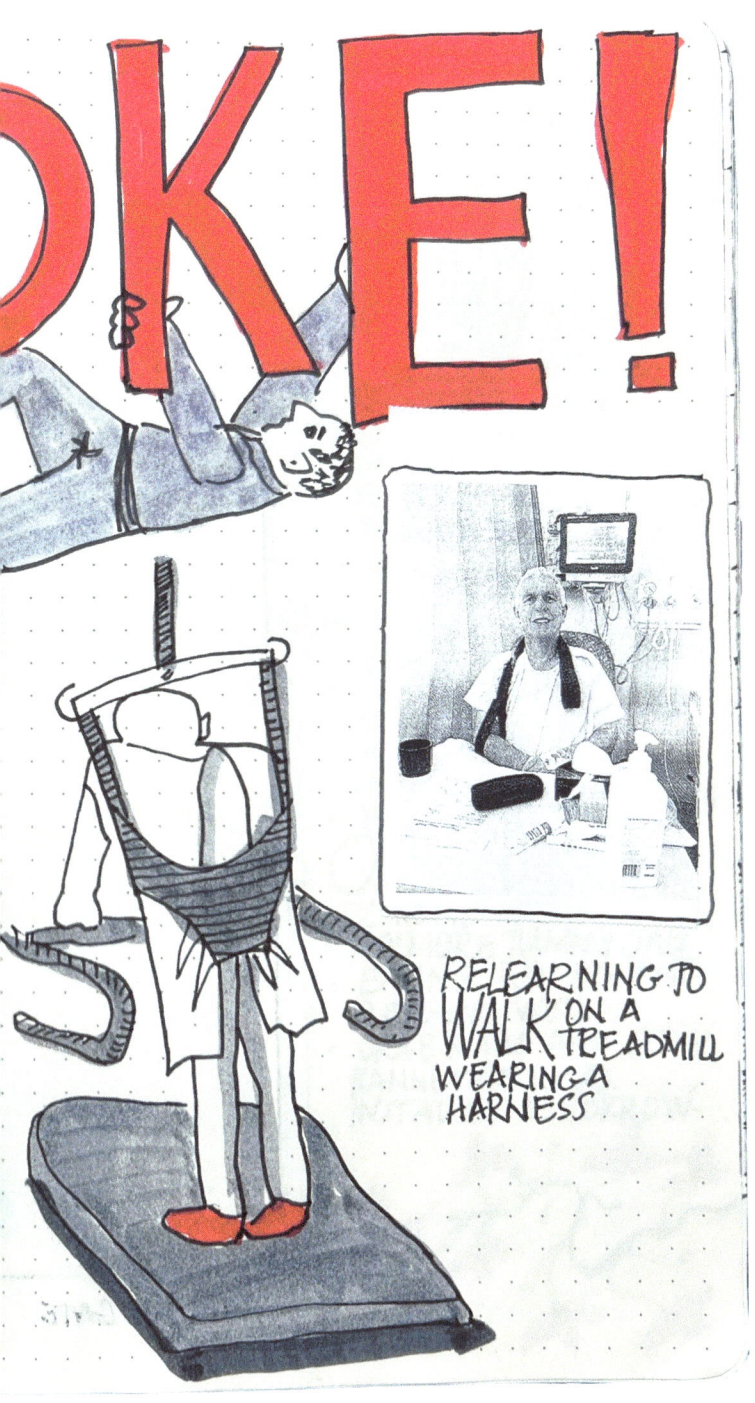

INTRODUCTION

In May 2023, I was struck down by a stroke losing movement to my right-sided limbs. This is the story of my recovery after that medical emergency. The content draws from actual writings and illustrations over a period of eighteen months.

Separated into three sections, Part One begins with daily messages, sent to family and friends, by Slobodanka (Bobby, my wife), in the first few weeks post-stroke. As witness to my brain assault, Bobby's words capture the real-time immediacy of disbelief and uncertainty surrounding the dramatic event that turned our lives upside down. Her writing is unedited to convey her thoughts, feelings and events as they unfolded.

In Part Two, I detail my physical recovery. First, in hospital and after that, as an outpatient, attending biweekly physiotherapy sessions, at the Brindabella Rehabilitation Centre ('Brindy'), at the University of Canberra Hospital. And living then, independently at home, as part of ongoing daily life. My recovery continues; it's an open-ended journey.

My candid writing style is an attempt to understand what had happened to me and to adapt to the altered state of my body. In my early reflections, my brevity is reflective of my compromised ability, as during the first few weeks I could only record my thoughts typing into my phone with one finger of my non-dominant left hand. I was unable to write as my right hand was lame. These physical limitations meant my writing style is reduced to short, single line sentences. As

I regained functional mobility, I progressed to typing with two or more fingers on my iPad before, months later, I recovered my full touch-typing ability, at slow pace. Writing, fluidly and steadily, with pen in hand, took longer to regain. Even now, writing by hand is slow.

Focus points, in this second section, coincide with key milestones and events as they occurred. For example, starting and completing my six-week 'Brindy' rehab program, and taking stock of my health at the sixth week, three- and six-month milestones. The more detailed accounts and flowing style are indicative of my growing dexterity, strength and stamina, along with greater clarity of mind and emotional stability.

In writing about these milestones there is some repetition, as the time gap between them, allowed for more reflection, bringing more coherence to understand how my body was responding to unfamiliar, and uncertain, circumstances. Rethinking the rehabilitation steps, akin to the repetitive daily exercise I had to do, for improving my strength, mobility and finer motor skills.

Bobby's drawings, taken from her illustrated journal of the time, contribute visually to this section. Many of the drawings she created while waiting for me to complete my two-hour physiotherapy sessions. Not being able to drive, I was dependent on her for getting to and from 'Brindy'.

Part Three features poetry and reflections of milestone events I wrote to sustain my mental and spiritual health as I continued with ongoing exercise for physical recovery. The poems inspired by sit spotting, a practice I learnt during an advanced ecotherapy course. I began the course nine months post-stroke and completed it in September 2024. The conclusion of this course is the end point to bring closure to this book.

Sit spotting is a practice of sitting quietly and comfortably outdoors to observe nature through full sensory awareness. The majority of my sit spot sessions have taken place around sunrise, or early morning, in my front garden. Other sessions at different times and locations in, or away, from Canberra, my home base.

I wrote most of my poems after sit spotting—hours, sometimes days after—to capture the sensory awareness and insights absorbed from being present in nature. Written in a minimalist and attentive style, they record observations within my being and outside in nature, as steps in my recuperation to balance body, mind and spirit. The poems record direct sensory experience; they are not streams of consciousness.

The creative and spiritual practice of writing poetry embodies my sensory experience of being grounded with nature, universal spirit and to myself. To nurture feelings of belonging, an important anchoring, when faced with the ongoing challenge of physical recovery, through repetitive exercise, while having to stay steady emotionally.

The seasonal changes of nature are apparent in my poetry and provide a cyclical, rather than a linear passage of time, which is more supportive of holistic healing.

The Future chapter brings the book to a close. I reflect on the factors that contributed to my post-stroke rehabilitation, enabling me to return to living with greater appreciation and better equipped to deal with life's challenges.

Part one
Day one to twenty-two

Bobby's daily email updates to family and friends.

DAY ONE

Tuesday, 2 May 2023

I'm sorry to let you know that this morning Thomas had a stroke, or at least a mini-stroke. He called me from Harrison saying he wasn't feeling well: confused, sweaty, pins and needles in his arm; slurring speech; dizzy, and generally crook. I took him to Calvary Hospital immediately. They were wonderful and conducted all sorts of tests. The CT brain scans were inconclusive as they could see no sign of bleeding or clots. But they decided to put him on blood thinning medication and monitor him for the next 24 hours as all the signs pointed to a stroke.

We will know more tomorrow. I'll stay in touch. I don't know what my movements will be over the next few days.

DAY TWO

Wednesday, 3 May 2023

I was at the hospital this morning but unable to sit with Thomas as they're still not sure if he has Covid or not. Came home to collect a few things and will go back again. I think he will be there for at least 4 days and then onto rehab somewhere. I'm guessing I'll not be back at work this week, but possibly next. He's very emotional today—understandably—and cannot move his right arm much nor grip with it. Also weakness in his right leg. They're going to try and stand him up this afternoon so we'll see how that goes.

* * *

Sadly, he's lost the use of his right arm and hand: can't grip anything. Also, some strength loss in right leg. Physio got him up and standing today but it's clear Thomas is going to have to relearn to walk. It's really a tragedy; very sad. I think he'll stay in hospital for a few more days and then if possible, they will transfer him to University of Canberra Hospital rehabilitation centre. Thomas is not keen and wants to be outpatient as he wants to come home, but I don't think that will be up to him to decide if he cannot walk. Early days: no forward planning. We're doing this one day at a time.

* * *

Thomas looked far better today, but during the course of the day his right-hand use deteriorated. He can't move it much and certainly cannot grip anything. His right leg is also affected. The physio came to get him up this afternoon and it is clear Thomas will have to relearn to walk again. He can't write, type or feed himself with his right hand. It's a tragedy.

The physio said more than likely they will transfer him to UC Hospital rehabilitation centre—once Thomas is stabilised—as an inpatient. Not as an outpatient. Thomas is of course dead set against this and says he wants to go home. Please, if you talk to him and he raises this, I hope you can persuade him that inpatient care would be the best for him initially.

But it's early days yet. By the time I left around 6.00 pm, we hadn't heard back from the revised Covid test—so I'm not sure when they will send him for an MRI scan. The affected hand bothered the doctor enough to ask for yet another CAT scan as they feared they may need to operate to insert a stent. You can imagine how that went down with Thomas. Luckily, they've decided to follow a conservative treatment plan: more blood thinners and fluids.

We'll see what tomorrow brings. This is very much one day at a time: no forward planning.

DAY THREE

Thursday, 4 May 2023

Thomas had a good day today. He looks better than yesterday and is speaking more. He enjoyed breakfast, which to his dismay included a bowl of baked beans, and lunch (lamb), which was interrupted by his being taken to have an MRI scan. The results of that will hopefully show where and what the stroke was.

Sadly, he cannot move his right hand and arm. His right leg is also weakened. But the physio got him walking (with assistance), which boosted Thomas's morale a whole heap. While she can't predict it accurately, she felt that Thomas would be able to walk unaided within about six months—if he continues in the same determined fashion. He also received electro-shock treatment to his muscles. These create movement, which mimics what he should be able to do with his hand—and aids the brain make new pathways of information. Once the hospital discharges him, we believe he will go to rehab at University of Canberra Hospital.

He is very emotional but says he wants to let out all the tears and frustrations so as not to impede physical progress. The staff are wonderful and Thomas is starting to joke with them—a very good sign. His speech is not as slurred, but he does have a droopy mouth on the right-hand side.

I'm fine but tired today as I didn't sleep well last night - stressing about what the future will bring. But I feel better after today. I was concerned because yesterday Thomas didn't want to go to rehab and was saying 'you can take me every day'! And my heart just sank because that would be so daunting. But today he's reconciled to going to rehab as an inpatient, which is so good.

DAY FOUR

Friday, 5 May 2023

Thomas made progress today. The speech pathologist cleared him to drink water out of a cup. This meant the fluids drip was removed and Thomas was freed from the pole and tubes.

The occupational therapist gave him 10 minutes of functional electrical stimulation, which enabled Thomas to grasp an object with his paralysed hand due to the muscles in his lower arm being stimulated. This is intended to encourage his brain to once again send messages to his hand.

With the help of three physiotherapists, Thomas walked 100 metres while supported (hanging from a harness) on a treadmill. This boosted his spirit and has given him hope that rehab will help him relearn to walk again.

The pastoral carer came to visit, which was good as Thomas was able to confirm that he is fine emotionally and doesn't want anti-depressants to numb his feelings.

He showered for the first time and shaved with his new electric razor. That certainly did him good. He's now set up with his iPhone, earplugs and Kindle to keep him company - although one is never alone in hospital. He enjoyed scrambled eggs for breakfast and macaroni cheese for lunch. I believe it's honey-soy chicken for dinner this evening.

The MRI scan has now proved conclusively that he had a stroke. The consultant spoke briefly to us late in the afternoon and said that she wants to keep Thomas in hospital for another 48 hours under observation and in care. The therapists have all reported that Thomas is an excellent candidate for the University of Canberra Hospital rehabilitation centre so the Calvary medical staff will engage with the rehabilitation staff for an interview with Thomas - and once there's a bed available, Thomas will move to this centre. We hope this will be in the course of next week. Once there, he will have at least 3 hours of rehab every day, plus access to the pool and their outdoor spaces - a boon for an outdoors man like Thomas.

DAY FIVE

Saturday, 6 May 2023

Thomas had a good day today: rest and reflection after a full four days of poking, prodding, testing, questioning and therapy. The hospital slows down on the weekend.

The best news is that it's likely he'll move to the rehab centre on Monday. I have to take him his civies: no slouching in pyjamas there! The clothes are in readiness for an early morning move. We hope this will be the case.

Other than that, Thomas is eating well, and his spirits are high - although he is still emotional, but that's fine. The hospital gave him a stroke information publication, which he read from cover to cover—and was quizzed on by a nurse. I'm pleased to say he passed the test with flying colours.

He told me this morning he did 5x5 repetitions of stepping up and down at his bedside - nothing if not determined to get back to walking. His right hand remains paralysed; we expect that it will take a while for his brain to relearn how to move that. He's going to settle in for dinner and a little TV tonight.

DAY SIX

Sunday, 7 May 2023

Thomas thanks you for all your care, good wishes and love. I've read him each message and email, which have given him huge support during these very challenging days.

Today was a good and relatively quiet day in hospital being a Sunday. The lovely Dr Sales visited Thomas and confirmed his transfer to UC Hospital rehabilitation centre.

I've packed his clothes so he's ready for an early transfer. But we understand this is dependent on there being a bed available. We are prepared for a local move to a less acute ward as an alternative. One day at a time.

Looking forward to a visit from Catherine (friend of Thomas) who is driving down from Mittagong. The snowstorm has slowed her down a little, but she's expected about 4.30 pm at Thomas's bedside.

DAY SEVEN

Monday, 8 May 2023

We enjoyed catching up with Catherine, who drew her own get-well card for Thomas. Enjoyed a visit from Louis who caught up with Thomas over lunch.

No move yet to rehab; still waiting for a bed.

Thanks everyone for all your messages of well-being directed at me. I'm taking your advice to look after myself with an early mark home. Just sitting back in the captain's chair enjoying the lovely autumn sunshine.

I've booked myself in for a medical this Wednesday - a checkup to make sure I'm functioning smoothly! Also taken up Louis's (Thomas' stepson) offer to speak to his colleague for an informal coffee and walk. Making sure my emotional makeup stays on track so I can focus my energy where it matters.

We hope Thomas will transfer tomorrow.

DAY EIGHT
Tuesday, 9 May 2023

We are in the super University of Canberra Hospital rehab centre. If you'd like to visit, Thomas is in the Stromlo ward, bed 5.

This morning the rehab transport was confirmed. Thomas put on his track pants and shoes in preparation. At noon, the wonderful ambulance staff arrived with a stretcher and just like that whizzed Thomas out of Calvary Hospital.

We are so grateful to the capable, conscientious, kind and qualified staff at the hospital. Every nurse, therapist, doctor, admin staffer and anyone else there was wonderful. Forever thankful.

At UC hospital, Thomas was immediately walked around the floor by another Thomas, the nurse. The facilities are top notch and Thomas is in a single room. That may change depending upon bed requirements. He may be moved to a 2-bed facility.

He was able to have a late lunch and is now napping. It's been a huge day. We expect a doctor round a little later but for the moment we're enjoying the peaceful premises.

Thank you everyone who say you like my updates; this is my form of therapy.

DAY NINE

Wednesday, 10 May 2023

Today rehab started in earnest. At 9.00 am Mel, the occupational therapist, interviewed Thomas. First to establish what are our home circumstances: five stairs from level 1 to level 2; shower and toilet accessibility; outdoor access—all of this in preparation for equipping the house with grab rails and bannisters. Then Mel asked Thomas to describe his milestones in order to go home. These range from being able to walk out of the hospital, hold a spoon in his right hand to feed himself, to being able to use toilets/bathrooms that don't have grab rails. After the interview, we moved to the gym.

The gym at UC Hospital is a very well used and equipped space that is full every day from 9-12 and again from 1-3. Each patient (and there are 30 in Stromlo where Thomas is) has their own personalised exercise regime.

Mel conducted an occupational assessment in order to set Thomas a series of exercises. These are as simple as gripping a spice jar, to doing bicep curls with his weak arm. He threw himself into all the tasks with energy and determination.

After occupational therapy, the student physiotherapist, Susanna, assessed Thomas's weak leg and walking ability. As with the occupational therapy, they will set Thomas a series of exercises to strengthen his floppy foot. The real regime starts in the morning.

After gym, we joined other patients in the communal sunny dining room for lunch. It's heartening to talk to residents who are happy to share their stories and provide encouragement to each other. After lunch, we retired to Thomas's room for a well-earned rest. He didn't have any other activities booked in so we explored the lovely internal courtyard garden (in a wheelchair) and rolled through the centre's passages and out the front door so that Thomas can orientate himself.

If you would like to visit, the best times are any weekday after 3.00 pm, Saturday afternoon and the whole of Sunday. Sadly, the cafe is not open over the weekends.

I hope you'll all be pleased to know that I visited my GP this morning for a health check: my blood pressure and heart are good. Next blood tests and more. Also had my Covid Booster No. 5 and anti-flu vaccination. Now back home with Bibi and Mr Bojangles. For the first day I'm feeling a little less tired and a little more content as Thomas is getting the BEST of care.

DAY TEN

Thursday, 11 May 2023

Today the silent patient Thomas has become the One Finger Poet. We're closing these 10 days of updates with Thomas's own words:

Stroke!

It came from nowhere
A silent peril
struck me
quickly
laid me low.

So unexpected
I'm fit, active, healthy, well.
What was it doing here, *inside me?*
In competent minds and caring hands
I landed.

Rapid Interventions
Infused with medication
monitoring around the clock
No pain

I can speak
I can think
I can swallow, eat and drink.

I feel . . . sad
mobility suspended, for now
I'm blessed
out of acute care
to rehab
allowed full, uninterrupted sleep.

Each day I build my strength
flexibility
oiling my joints through movement
repetitions
willing muscles to flex
twitch, respond.

Kindness
all around me.
Everyone focused on
my care.
So much support for Bobby, Louis and me.

If you're going to have a stroke, have it in Canberra!

Thomas wants me to thank you again for your messages, support and love. Now that he's in rehab and working hard in the gym, we hope to see many improvements. We will update again next week.

DAY ELEVEN

Friday, 12 May 2023

All going in the right direction, I hope. Thomas is getting lots of physio and occupational therapy. He can now grip my hand, which he couldn't do a few days ago. But this evening he was complaining of a bloated and bruised stomach—he's getting daily injections of something straight into his belly—so was upset by that. But reported it to the nurse so I hope he will be seen by a doctor this evening. There is a list of guests lined up to visit him over the course of this week. The OT said I could take him out over the weekend for a drive or to visit home. They've given me the name of someone who will be able to put in bannisters and grab rails in our house.

DAY TWELVE

Saturday, 13 May 2023

Thomas again as the One Finger Poet:

Repair

Lift
Lift
Lift

Repetitions

Raising weakened limbs
over
and over again.

Lift
Lift
Lift

Willing muscles to move
to respond

find their neural connection
to fire
and ignite familiar movement.

Lift
Lift
Lift

Repair . . .
through repetition
My body . . .
will it respond today?

Lift
Lift
Lift

DAY FOURTEEN

Monday, 15 May 2023

As you know, Thomas suffered a stroke on 2 May, which has radically shifted the ground under us both. But wonderful things happen as life, love and memory continue. I'm delighted to have worked with my dear friend Lorraine to produce her book, *We were all somebody else yesterday*. She's written an amazing account of her early life, short stories full of feeling, with equal parts of trauma and joy. This is a private publication for her family. It has inspired Thomas to continue writing his memoir, albeit with one hand. This gives him something to strive towards during rehabilitation.

DAY FIFTEEN
Tuesday, 16 May 2023

A fortnight ago Thomas had a stroke and our world changed. Since then, he's spent a week at Calvary Hospital. He was admitted via Emergency where the wonderful staff ran him through a series of tests and confirmed that he'd had a stroke caused by a blockage in the lower part of his brain. The effect of this was paralysis of his right arm and hand, and right foot with a weakened right leg. Thankfully Thomas can talk and has all his cognitive abilities - even telling jokes!

A week ago he was admitted to the University of Canberra Hospital Rehabilitation Centre. He will stay there until he is mobile enough and it is safe for him to return home. He's working out at the gym 3-5 hours every day. The physios and occupational therapist have set him a series of exercises to strengthen and get his limbs moving. Thomas is working as hard at these as if preparing for an ultra-marathon (he's run two).

The rehab centre is an excellent facility, purpose-built to assist patients to regain their mobility with dignity and in comfort. Thomas has a good appetite and enjoys his meals in the dining room, chatting with other patients. He's very busy throughout the day and if you want to visit, please do so after 3.00 pm. It's lovely sitting in the internal courtyard enjoying a cup of tea with him.

We decided it would be good for me to return to work—now that we know he is safe and comfortable and working hard himself—so I'm WFH in the mornings. In the afternoons I visit Thomas where we have a good chat about all his activities and I fill him in on mine. We're looking to make the house safe for him by adding grab rails and bannisters on the stairs. Thomas was even allowed to go out over the weekend so we drove home. He sat on our verge bench enjoying the sun, patting Bibi and Bobo who came to say hello. It's these little pleasures that sustain him going forward.

DAY TWENTY

Sunday, 21 May 2023

I feel

*A filigree of fear
Under a crusted lace carapace.
It cloaks my
Forcing fingers through
the sharpness
Of blinding white gauze.*

Bobby Graham

DAY TWENTY-TWO

Tuesday, 23 May 2023

Thomas has been discharged from University of Canberra Hospital rehab centre - at least as an inpatient. He can come home tomorrow after two weeks of rehab and remediation. From Thursday, he starts again as an outpatient, going to UC Hospital 3 or 4 times a week for rehab at the Brindabella Centre.

He's made good progress with mobility and strength and is now able feed himself with his right hand. He can make a fist, grip a small object, pick it up, and tap most of his fingers with his thumb.

The next frontier is his foot, which he is coaxing into movement and flexibility. He is able to walk unaided, climb stairs unaided and negotiate a grassy slope unaided. We've had the house fitted with grab rails and bannisters - just in case. The biggest exercise now is patience!

We'd like to thank the enthusiastic, helpful, kind and skilled staff at the University of Canberra Hospital rehab centre, Stromlo Ward. They have been unfailingly cheerful and supportive, not only to Thomas, but to all the patients in their care. It's an amazing centre and we are very fortunate in Canberra to have access to this facility.

So, from tomorrow we look forward to the next steps!

Part two
Post-stroke recovery: physical

We now switch from Bobby's experience, during the first three weeks, to my reflections of this period and subsequent key milestones in my ongoing rehabilitation.

DAY FIFTEEN

Tuesday, 16 May 2023

Stromlo Unit, University of Canberra Rehabilitation Hospital

An arm and a leg

My dominant side is my right side.

With my right arm and leg, I accomplished so much.

My right hand held a knife at meals. Could throw a dart accurately. Cup a handful of water beside a stream.

Hold a spade when gardening. A leash when walking Bibi, our pet fox terrier, around Yerrabi Ponds.

The steering wheel when driving the ute as Mr Petman.

Hold a pen to write, to sign my name. To extend a hand in greeting.

To stroke Bojangles, my cat. Bowl a ball to Louis. Cuddle Bobby.

My right leg transported me in ultra marathons, up Chapman's Peak and Constantia Nek during the Two Oceans.

Supported me when hiking outback trails—Kakadu, Walls of Jerusalem and the coastal Tarkine.

My right leg and foot could curve a ball from the corner post into the goal square with ease when playing soccer.

Hold a rhythmic beat on the dance floor.

My legs allowed me to walk, amble, jog, run, cycle and swim.

These limbs held and supported life, embraced life.

Dexterous, flexible, so strong and versatile.

They're more than limbs—they are a vital part of me.

Their complete dependability, suddenly interrupted by a stroke. I need to recapture and rebuild their functional attributes.

A week ago, my arm was lifeless—a dead 10kg weight.

It's amazing how heavy a non-functioning arm is. My hand unresponsive.

My leg was better, though weak with a floppy, lazy foot.

A team of physiotherapists are devising rehabilitation exercises for me and guiding me through the routines.

They're all young, bright and highly skilled.

Mel, the senior, she's the assessor and strategist.

Learning about my home setting, to eliminate any obstacles, for when I return.

And designing exercises to stimulate the various muscles in my arm, before handing over to Emily who wires me up to FES devices to send electric pulses to my hand, miraculously bringing it to life.

And manual exercises to flex my wrist, move my forearm and unclasp my fingers.

Through repetitive movement, I seek to find the smallest sign of life, willing myself to move unresponsive muscles.

The slightest twitch a win. One twitch, two, three, four . . .

To get the hand functional, we're starting with the shoulder muscles, working down my arm to the elbow, then wrist, to the hand.

The muscles around each joint need to be exercised independently.

Working through mini exercises, often with the help of my good left arm, electrical stimulation or being rigged to pulleys on a rehab bench, my muscles are encouraged to move.

It's hard work willing, breathing, thinking life into muscles that have lost their natural neural pathways.

Briana, a physiotherapist, is devising strength-building exercises for both my arm and leg, passing me onto Susanna, the enthused fourth year physiotherapist student, who puts me through the routines.

I aim for quality repetitions, in cycles of 25.

Susanna is keen, caring—a benevolent whip cracker, egging me on. EFFORT. Yes, CAPITAL EFFORT, brings positive rewards—movement, strength, sensation.

Five hours a day, including one hour on my own.

In the day, I join about 30 others in the shared therapy gym—10m x 25m—where all the workstations are alive with bodies under active repair. A mixed gender bag aged from 50s to 95—no young people.

My arm is regaining life. I feel it in the shoulder. I can sense it once again, the muscles, even tone. It's a good feeling.

I can open my hand, move my fingers. Have a motion to grasp.

And so it is with leg and foot. From this morning, I was allowed to walk unaided.

At 5.00 am I appeared like a ghost from my room, startling the nurses, as I began to walk laps of the corridors.

More than a kilometre, with a staggered gait. A start. A good start.

I'm lucky to be here. I'm in good hands.

An arm and a leg—a simple arm and a leg, I see them differently now.

Patience needs to be my friend.

One finger patient

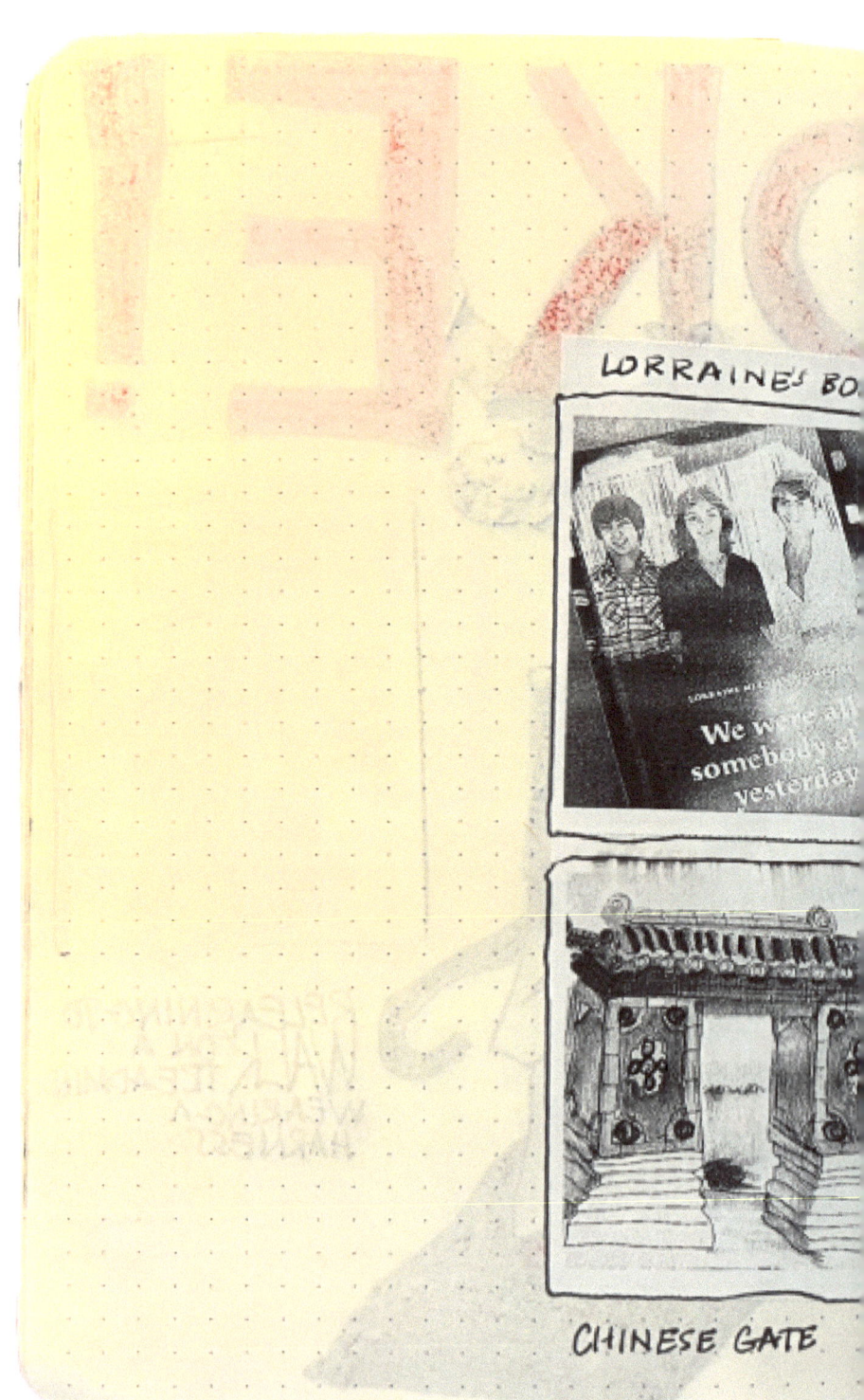

MONDAY
22 MAY

NEARLY 3 WEEKS POST STROKE

THOMAS HAS MADE MASSIVE PROGRESS. ONE WEEK IN CALVARY TWO WEEKS AT UNIVERSITY OF CANBERRA HOSPITAL REHAB. WITH BRIAN A AND SUSANNA HIS PHYSIOS HE IS RE-BUILDING.

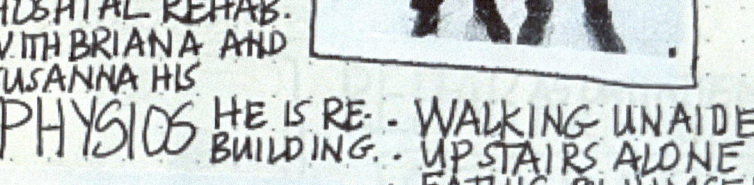

- WALKING UNAIDED
- UPSTAIRS ALONE
- EATING BY HIMSELF GRIPPING A SPOON IN HIS RIGHT HAND.
- SHOWERING ALONE.
- WRITING POETRY WITH ONE FINGER
- 2 HOME VISITS
- NO MORE TUMMY JABS
- EATING, POO-ING AND SLEEPING WELL
- GRAB RAILS AND STAIR BANNISTERS TO BE INSTALLED TOMORROW.

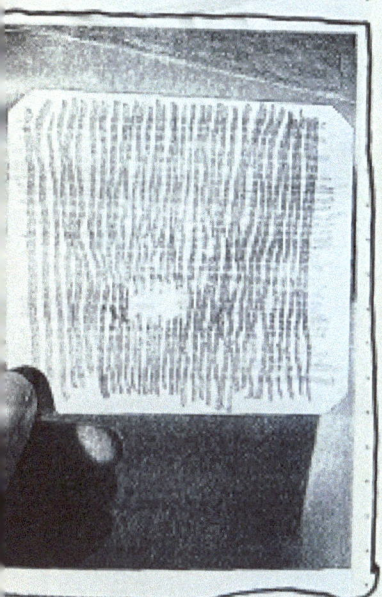

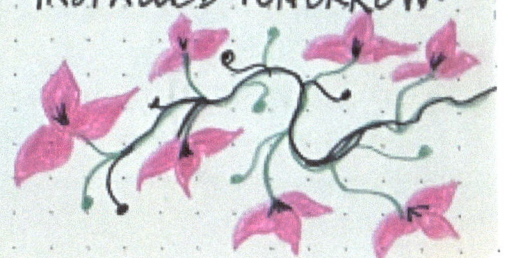

DAY TWENTY-THREE

Wednesday, 24 May 2023

My first day at home after being released from rehab hospital

The power to heal

The mind, body and spirit work together in repair.

Laid low by a stroke, I was lucky to keep most of my mobility and cognitive faculties, though my right arm and leg were badly affected.

The arm reduced to a dead weight held in a supportive sling, its muscles little more than jelly, weak and non-responsive.

The hand clasped closed, the fingers immobile.

My leg was better but not the foot. With help I could stand, with support on either side. I could step forward slowly, my leg and foot a wobbly uncoordinated duo, as if unknown to each other.

It was a shock to have lost full, functioning and flexible movement I'd known, relied upon and embraced all my life.

For the first time in 66 years, familiar movement wasn't there. Paradoxically, it had gone walkabout, out of immediate reach.

I could no longer stand on my own two feet, unaided.

My natural, confident stride, strong and controlled—absent.

This realization hit me hard. Confronting, as being movement compromised wasn't part of my known world, nor what I desired.

How to think?

Where to turn?
Who to rely on?
Is there a when?
What to do?

Get up and move.

Get up and take that first step. Try, will, imagine one finger moving.

Elyse and Emma—physiotherapist and occupational therapist respectively—got me up on day one. 'Let's go for a walk', Elyse invited.

My first healing agents—angels perhaps—they delivered hope for repairing my body.

Getting me to think about familiar body movements.

They believed my non-responsive limbs could function again, even when witnessing their wasted, weak and fragile state.

My limbs did not always respond when I wanted, willed and begged them to.

When they didn't move, Elyse and Emma offered calm, unwavering encouragement. They made me exercise, got me on my feet. Stimulated my hand with electrical charges.

As my self-doubt wrestled with self-belief, they were all I had—along with a few Hail Mary's.

I wept at my loss.

The doctors offered anti-depressants. NO! I don't want to be numbed. I want to feel, to express my emotions. I have every reason to be sad. Let me feel. To regroup, to understand what has happened to me.

My tears were most often out of relief, not grief—as I was grateful for so much—my speech, my functioning mind, my ability to swallow, eat and drink, my remaining able limbs, intact, mobile and strong. For the care and kindness that surrounded me.

For the support given to Bobby and Louis who suffered their own shock and disbelief—they had only ever known me as energetic, mobile, fit and healthy.

What had happened to Thomas?

The effect on them, paralleled my own afflicted limbs and hospitalization, to monitor the aftershocks of what may come next.

To everyone who sent Bobby, Louis and I texts, emails, FB posts, handwritten cards or letters; who made a telephone call, sent flowers, offered prayers, brought gifts to the door, visited me in hospital or completed tasks I could not complete—I thank you.

Friendships along with hope, belief and exercise, brought balm to bathe my damaged limbs, helped soothe my unsettled emotions and delivered comfort to Bobby and Louis.

They lifted us up.

In moments of shock and uncertainty, being remembered is wonderfully uplifting.

The support for Bobby was amazing as she bore witness to virtually every key moment—admission to the emergency ward, being given clot-busting medication, scanned, first shuffling steps, initial electrically stimulated hand movements, limbs suspended by pulleys engaged in repetitions, treadmill walks at snail's pace, one-handed meals, seated showers, bedside chats.

On the seventh day, I was transferred to rehab hospital, a short ambulance trip down the road.

To a new team of healing agents, doctors, occupational practitioners and physiotherapists, Mel, Emily, Briana and Susanna—all focused on my recovery.

The daily routine to get me, to get my limbs, responsive to movement again.

At 9 am each morning—Sunday excluded—I've pitched up at the shared therapy gym to begin active exercise of arm and leg.

Four to five hours a day and more, at my bedside, in the early hours of the morning and at night.

A twitch or slightest stir of movement the first sign of life. A point from which to start recovery.

With each passing day strength, movement and sensation slowly returned to affected areas. Each progression an incentive to do more.

Within a couple of days, I was allowed to walk and shower unaided. I gave up the wheelchair to take ungainly steps between my room, the gym, dining room and outside courtyards.

At 5 am, I paced the corridors, notching up precious metres to strengthen my leg, to reaffirm my balance and experience my body in motion. I could walk!

Functional Electric Stimulation (FES) helped to open my unresponsive hand, miraculously, allowing me to exercise the fingers. Other manual exercises freed the wrist and pulling on therabands ignited the muscles up and down my arm, bringing them back to life.

To dispense with the arm sling, my shoulder muscles had to be stronger, so that I could outstretch my right arm at 90 degrees from my body, and hold it there, for at least two seconds. Sounds simple but when your muscles are jelly, it ain't.

After several days of exercise, I could ditch the sling, giving greater flexibility to move both arms in tandem. To aim for balance, my right side mimicking my left side. The tactile sensation of clasping two hands together or rubbing the palms of my hands against my naked thighs, a blissful comfort.

Regaining regular movement—slow, weak and shaky—signaled reconnection. The brain and body learning new neural pathways for limbs to function again. Neuroplasticity in practice. The body repairing itself through belief, mind imaging and by watching my movements in a mirror.

For seventeen consecutive days, Bobby came to the hospital to watch my progress.

A COVID outbreak in the ward brought a halt to all visitations. I, along with other patients, were confined to our rooms. No visitors and no formal gym. A temporary setback.

I continued to exercise in my room and on my bed. The small mobility gains building self-belief. My body, weak yet responsive, was coming back to life.

It had taken a battering.

The physical trauma of the stroke had killed a small area of my brain, the clot blocking vital oxygen to my head.

A physical assault of medical interventions followed to determine the cause, type and location of the stroke along with high doses of medications, and frequent monitoring, to reduce any likelihood of an immediate reoccurrence.

I also had to adjust to the hospital environment, designed to support my recovery but by its nature, putting additional strains and stresses on my body.

The hot air-conditioned ward dried my eyes, nose and throat—I'm a fresh air man.

Most often the lights were on, making sleep and rest difficult under the harsh artificial light.

My movement restricted by intravenous lines inserted into my veins feeding nutrients to my body and cables stuck to my chest monitoring my heart.

And the constant monitoring of my vital signs—consciousness, blood pressure, temperature, oxygen levels and heart beats—day and night.

Being in an acute ward, with other patients, there was little down-time as nurses and doctors did their rounds around the clock, pushing their COWs (Computer on Wheels) ahead of them to take readings or to input data.

The care and attention were outstanding, the nurses vigilant, skilled and friendly. A mix of Australian-born and new Australians drawn from across the globe: India, Nepal, Fiji, Nigeria, Ethiopia,

Bhutan, South Africa, China, Philippines and Tonga. Without exception, highly trained, courteous and kind.

My first couple of weeks were a blur of sensory experiences forcing the body and mind to adapt to the trauma of the stroke, loss of mobility, intense medical interventions, the hospital environment and the unknown of what recovery would look like.

It was scary stuff adjusting to a reality I'd never experienced before.

A major plus was being free of pain. The one inconvenience having a blood thinning injection in my abdomen each morning. The injection bloated my tummy and caused much bruising as if I'd been pummeled black and blue.

Dealing with uncertainty lead to reflection and writing. I was fortunate my entry to the rehab hospital coincided with a pilot workshop about poetry and wellbeing led by Dr Owen Bullock, a University of Canberra lecturer.

I joined other patients at the hour-long, once a week class, with a heightened need to express myself, as similar to my fellow participants we'd all lost something of ourselves. Despite the excellent care, we were all seen primarily as patients, not as whole individuals.

Many felt they'd lost their vital spirit, their humanity diminished, without a private space to retreat to. Our rooms—single or shared—were not our own personal spaces, but primarily communal workspaces we shared with staff. We all experienced a tension with this duality and one evening, Owen asked us to write about it.

My contribution, typed on my phone with one finger, took about ten minutes:

Private spaces

I'm allocated a room.
In fact, a bed,
Stromlo Unit, Bed 5.

It's my sanctuary.
My private space
To sleep, eat and wash.
To rest.
To get to know this new person
I've become.

And then they move me.

I keep my bed—it has wheels,
But lose my room
It wasn't mine after all.
Someone else needed it.

I'm moved into shared digs
Bed 13, next to Bed 14,
The space divided by a curtain.

Do I dig in
or wait until
I'm wheeled to another room?

I'm not at home,
I'm in rehab hospital.

Take me home
To my own bed and room,
To my bed without wheels.

The poetry writing sessions were a soothing getaway to temporarily settle into a different headspace, to deal with the damage inflicted on our bodies, as well as adjusting to institutional care. We all left buoyed by being able to express ourselves creatively.

I made a point of being friendly with the nursing staff, who as I mentioned were kind, considerate and empathetic. Amiena, a nursing aide, I discovered hailed from Cape Town originally, migrating to Australia in the very year we had and was living in the same suburb we did. Not only that—she could make *koeksisters* and *samoosas*!!

One weekend, when I was allowed out on a day pass, to escape the ward lockdown—Bobby and I tucked into Amiena's freshly baked authentic Cape Malay *koeksisters*. *Lekker*!

Today, 22 days post-stroke, I was discharged from rehab hospital to transition into outpatient care. I came home, to Bobby, Bojangles, Bibi and my bed without wheels.

Over future weeks, I will return to the Brindabella Centre, the outpatient rehabilitation unit at the hospital, to continue intensive physio.

My recovery is going well, my initial goals were to walk out of the hospital and feed myself, to hold a spoon in my affected hand.

I did both this morning, way quicker than anticipated due to consistent hard work and determination aided by my therapists—I could not have done it without them. Nor without Bobby, who has sat by my side, calmly egging me on.

I walked out of the hospital this morning, not heroically triumphant, but in humble appreciation of the power of my body to heal itself, inspired by a suite of encouraging therapists.

I may not have been a typical target for a stroke with regard to risk factors, but the health and wellbeing of my body before the stroke has certainly expedited my recovery.

I'm not getting ahead of myself.

I still have much body repair to do—my right leg has regained about 60% of its strength, the foot and ankle about 75% of their dexterity and flexibility; my right arm has got back 50% of its strength and about the same in nimbleness and finer motor skills.

My hand and fingers are fully functional though remain weak—I need to strengthen further arm muscles so I can write and use tools again.

The rest of my body is 100% fit and strong.

It's a comforting and inspirational base to work from.

Over the next three weeks I will go all out with rehab exercises to return my remaining strength and functionality before reassessing my physical abilities once more.

I want to drive, hike, jog, swim, write and type normally again.

The mind, body and spirit have worked in unison to facilitate repair.

Neuroplasticity works!

Tomorrow, I begin another phase towards full recovery.

Stroke survivor

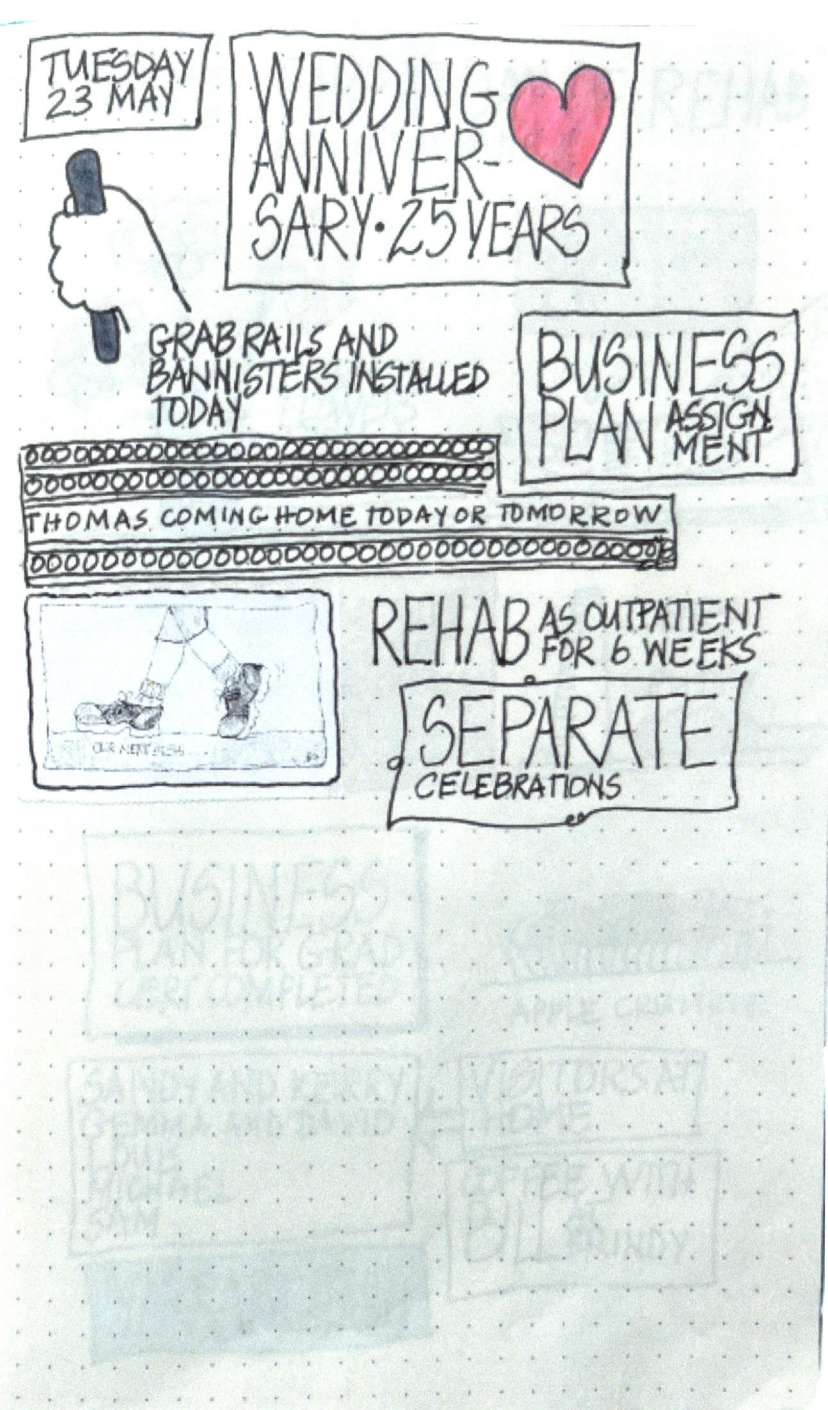

TUESDAY 23 MAY

WEDDING ANNIVERSARY · 25 YEARS ♥

GRAB RAILS AND BANNISTERS INSTALLED TODAY

BUSINESS PLAN ASSIGNMENT

THOMAS COMING HOME TODAY OR TOMORROW

REHAB AS OUTPATIENT FOR 6 WEEKS

SEPARATE CELEBRATIONS

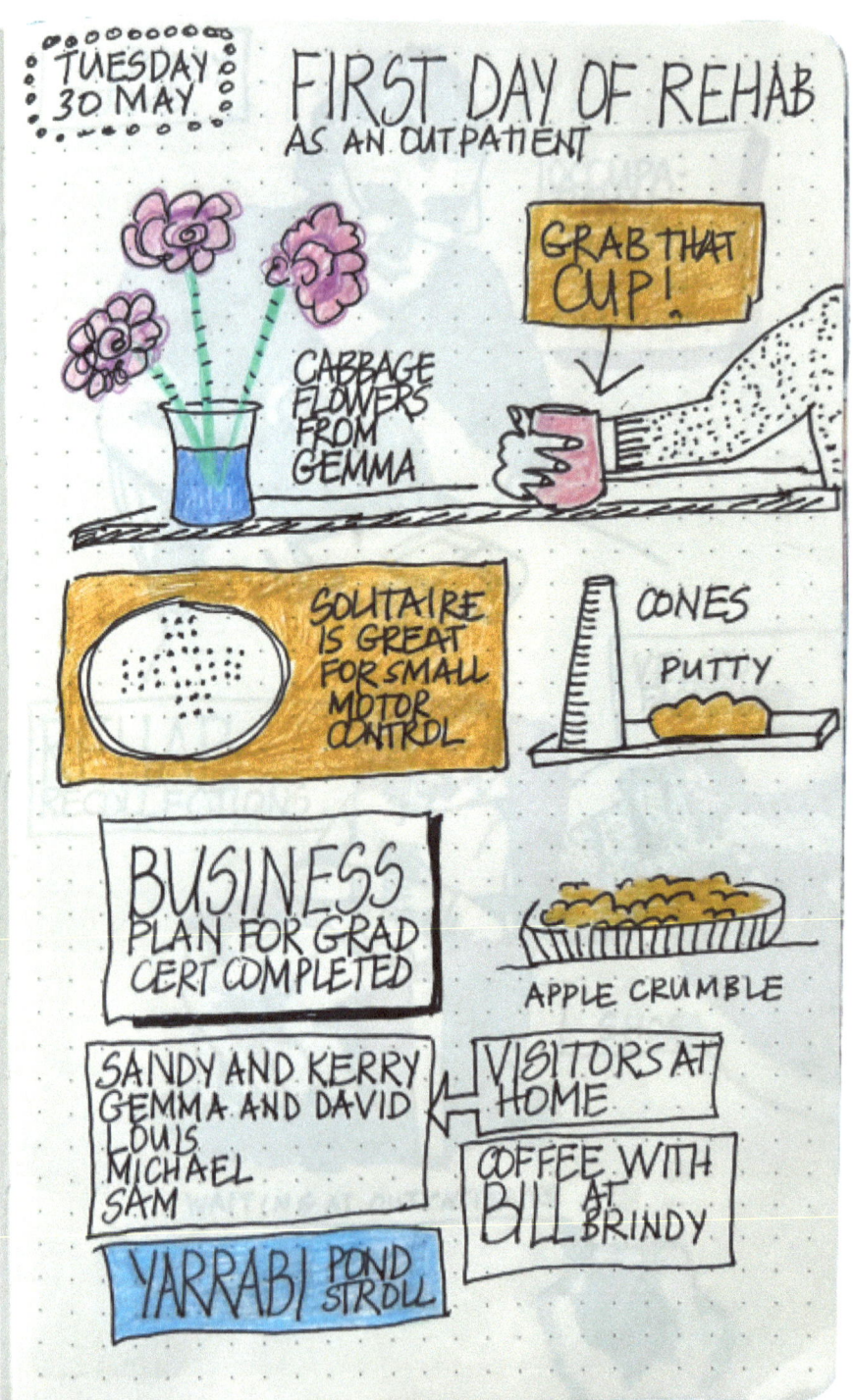

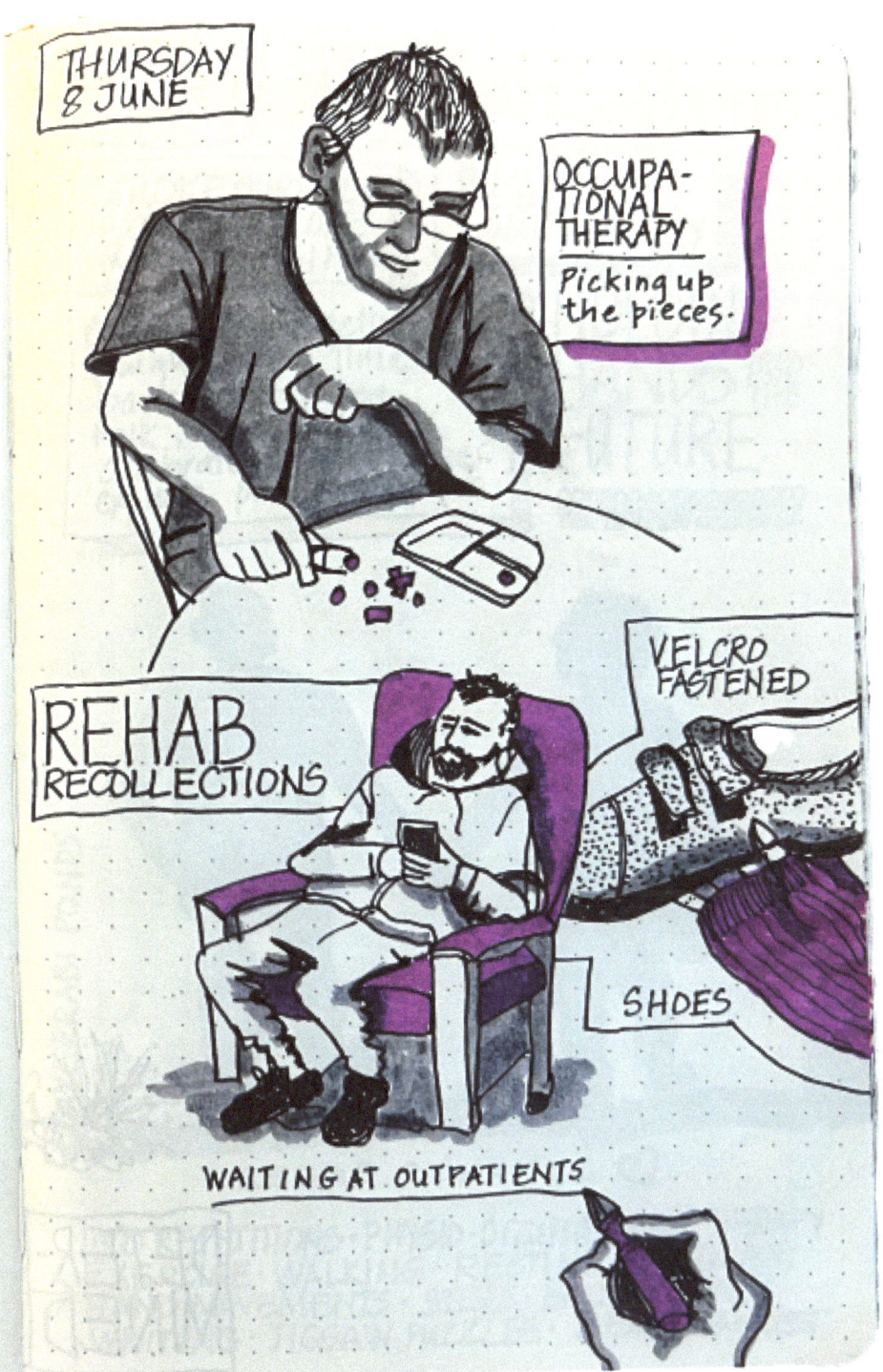

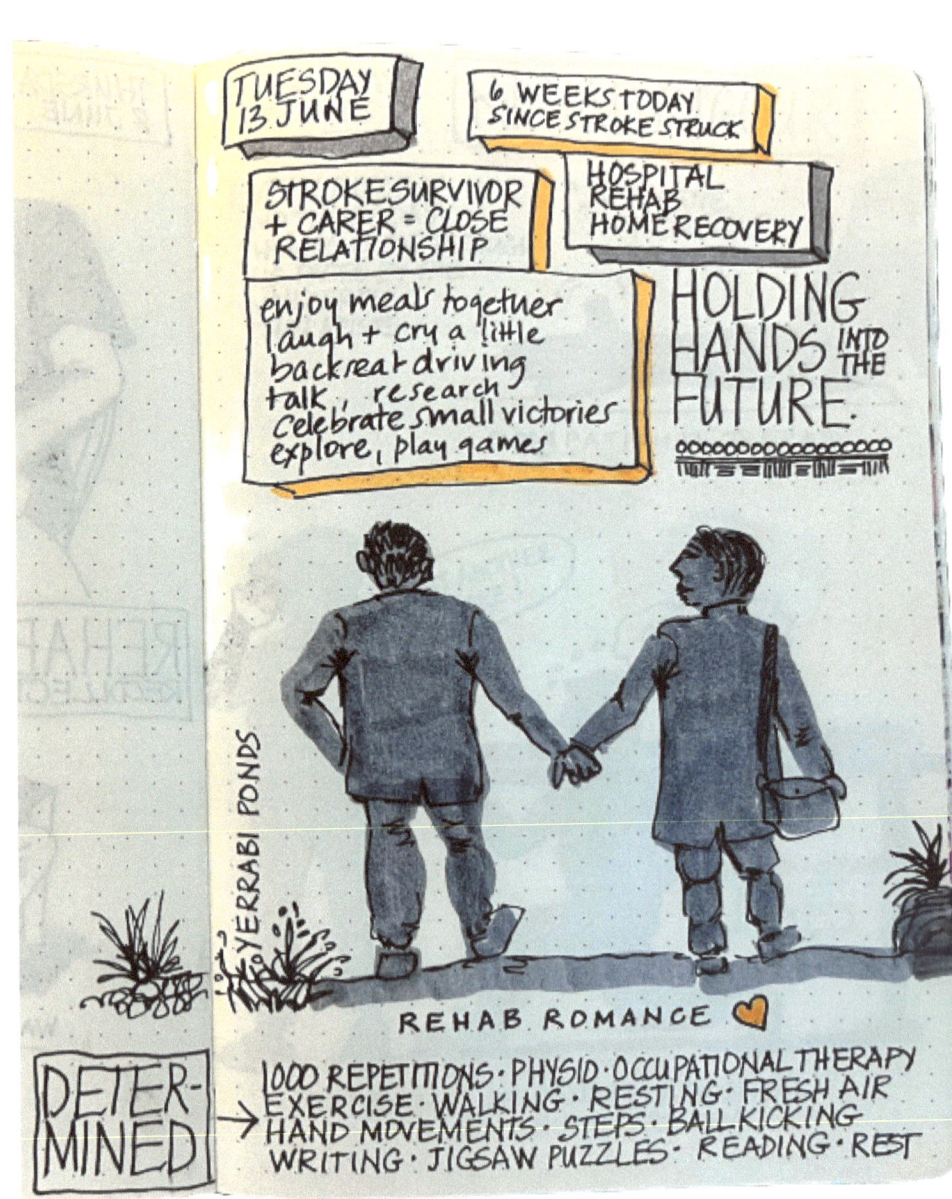

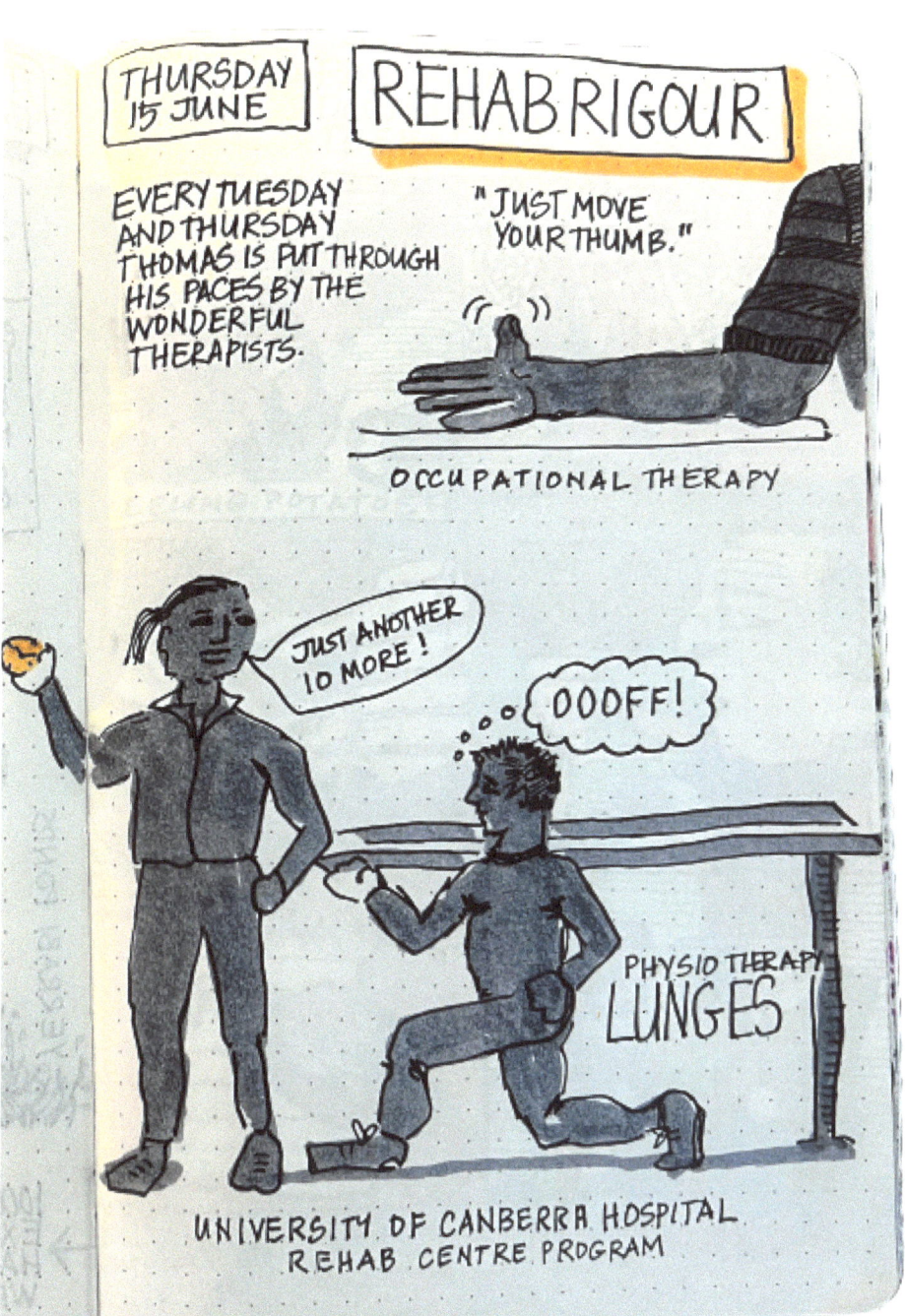

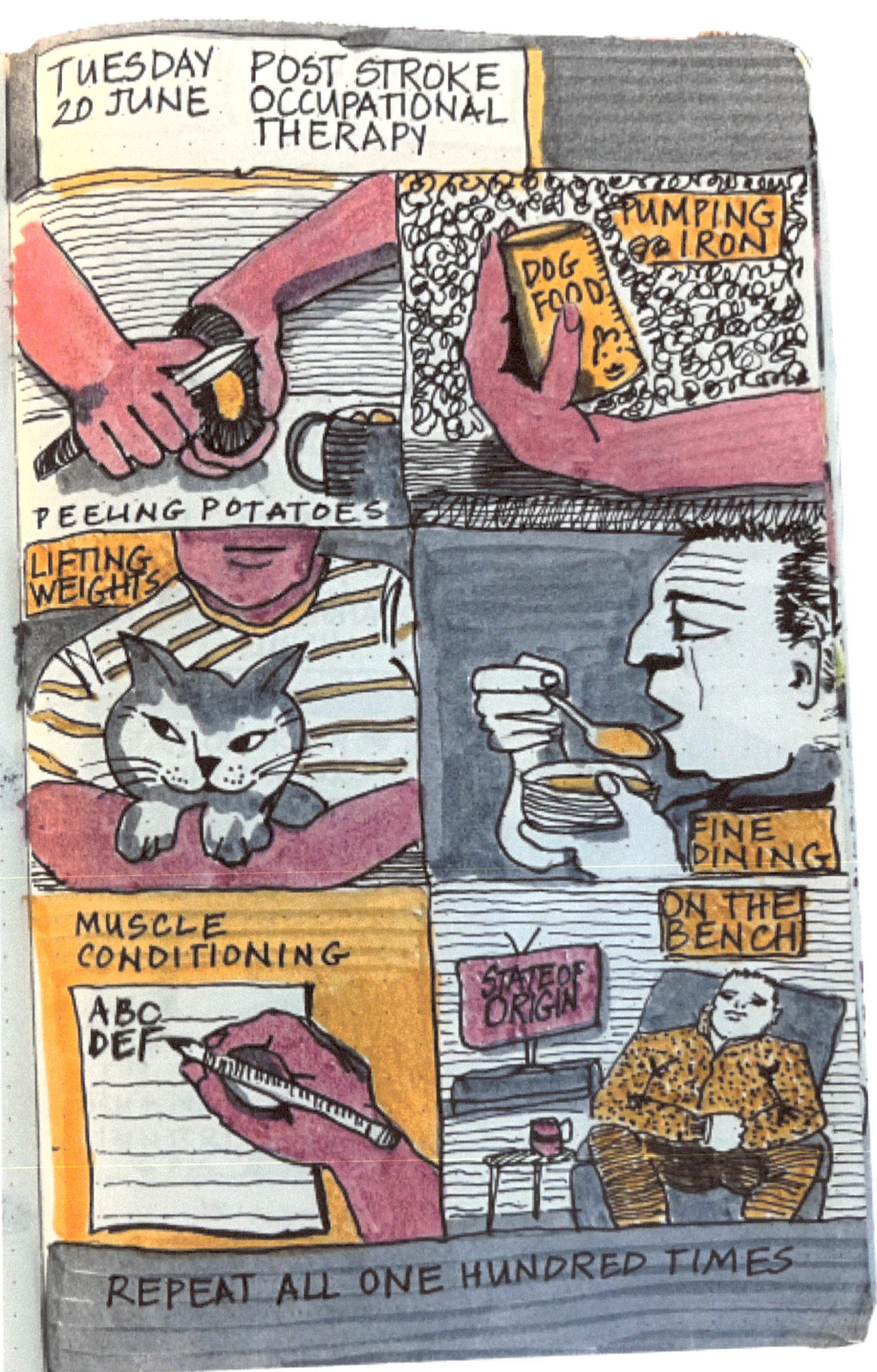

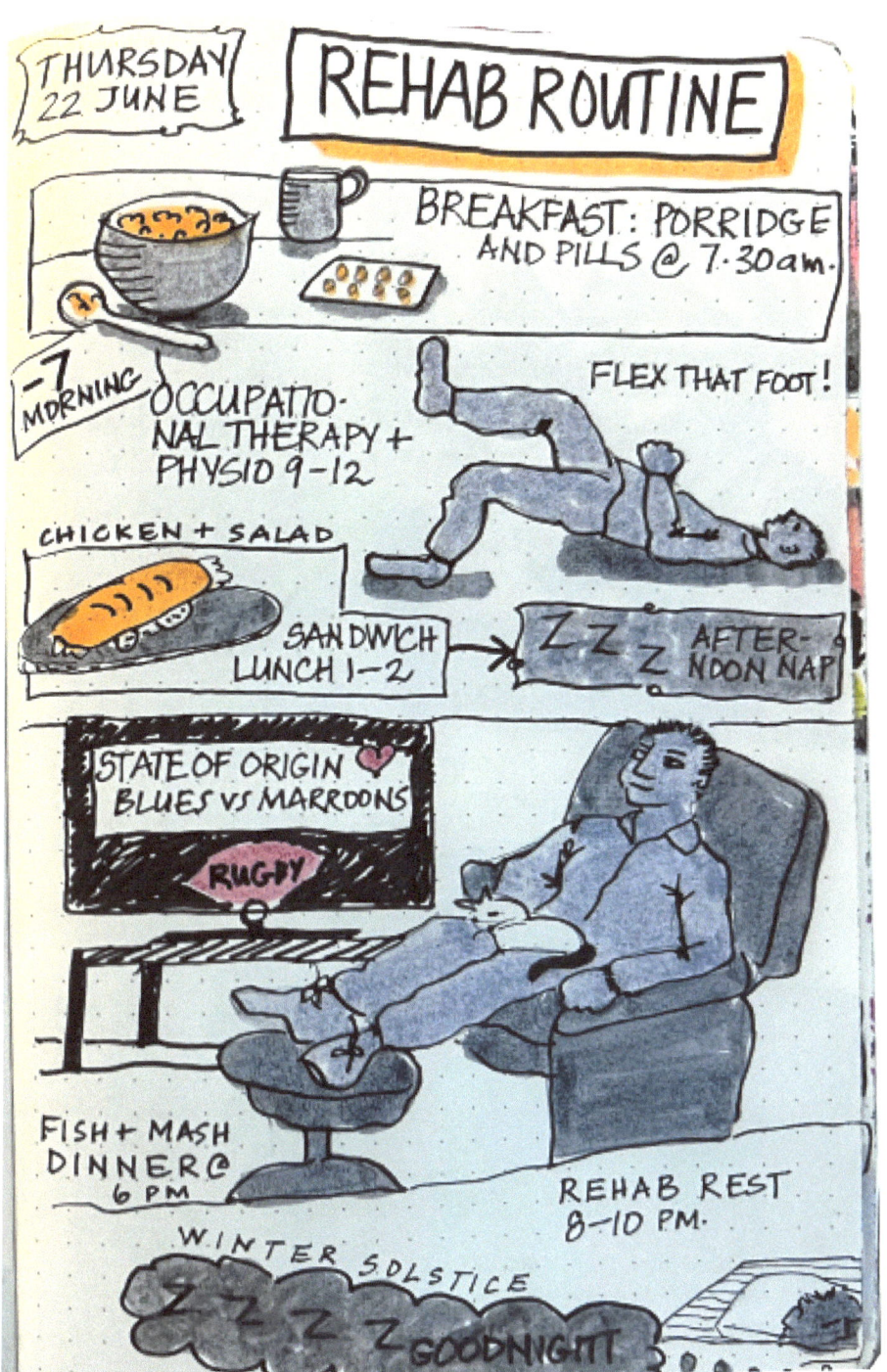

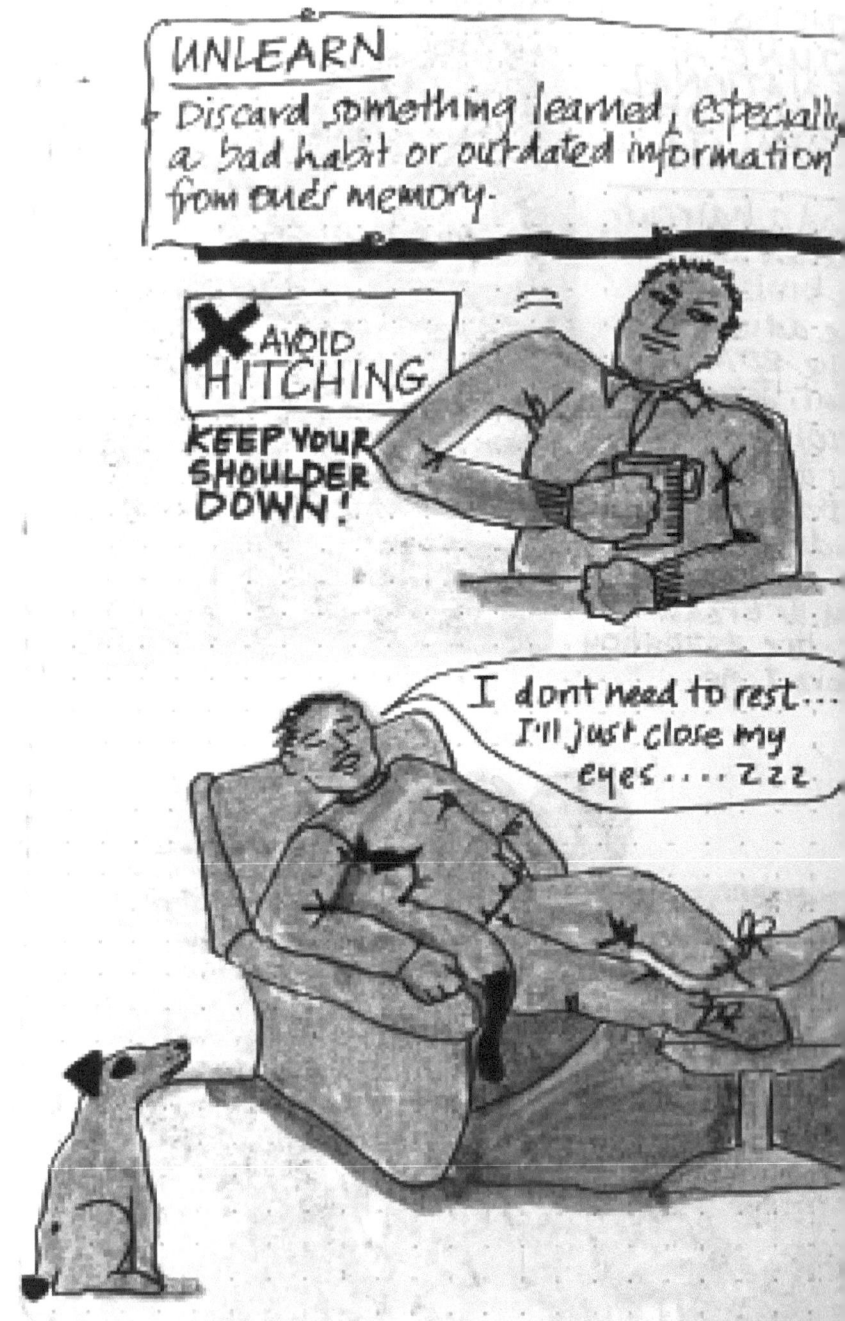

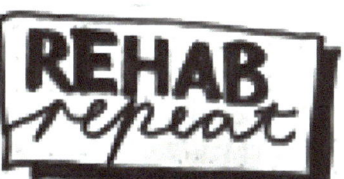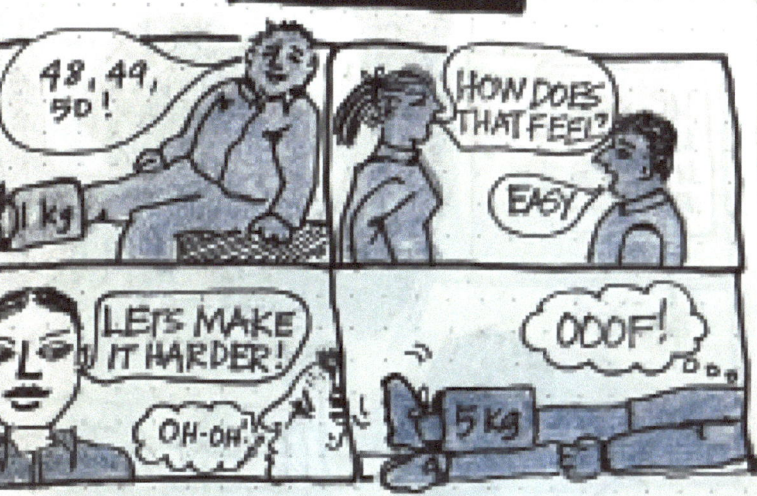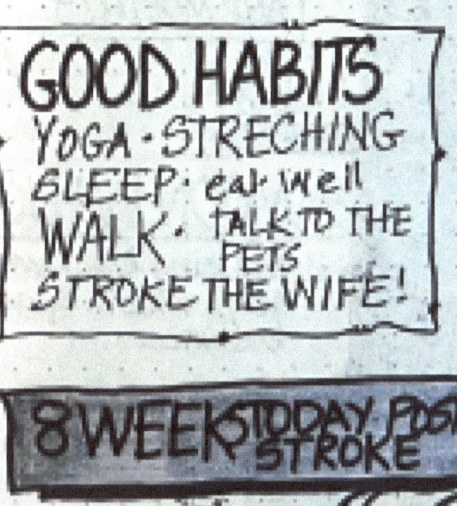

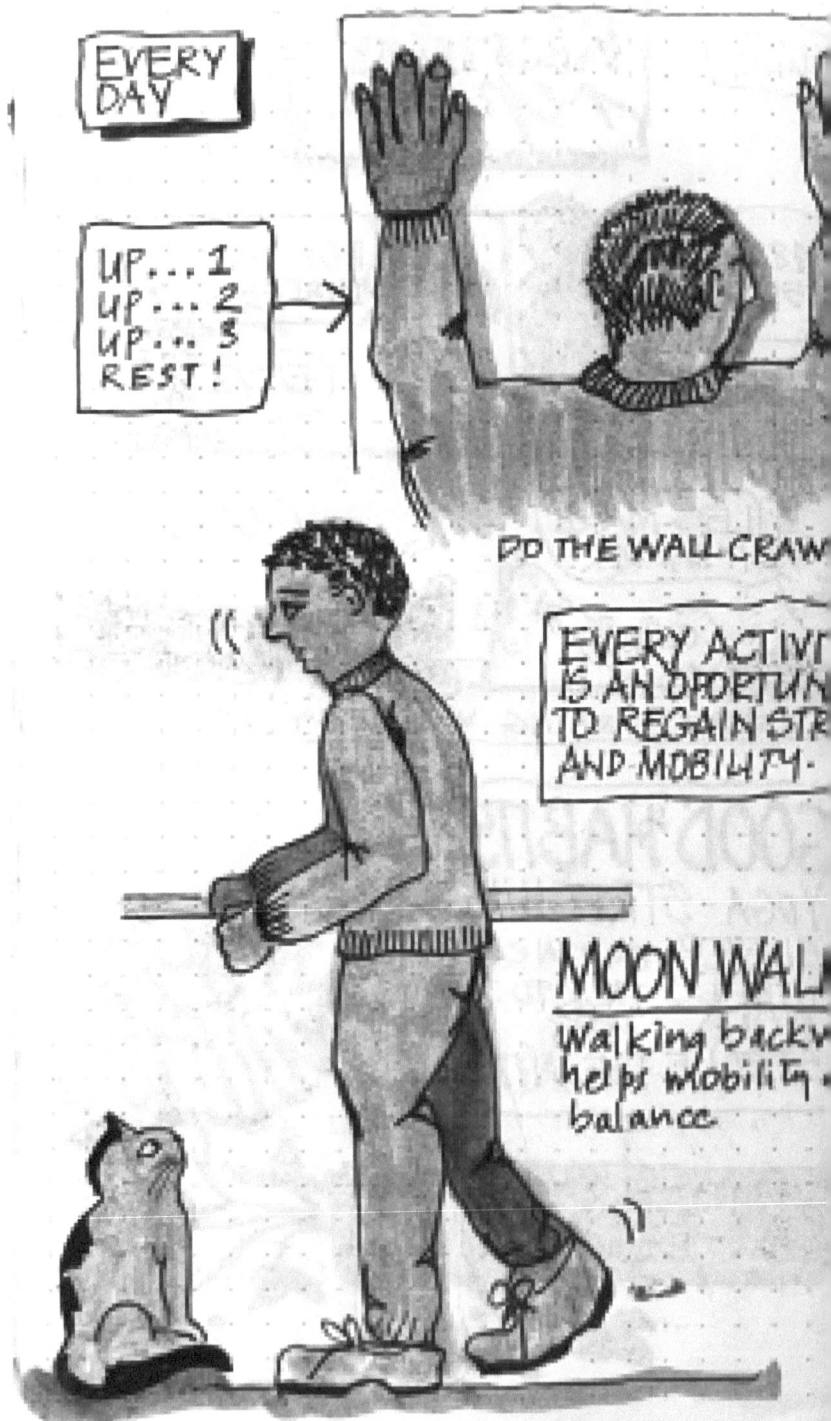

THURSDAY
24 JUNE

"RAPID" REHAB GAINS

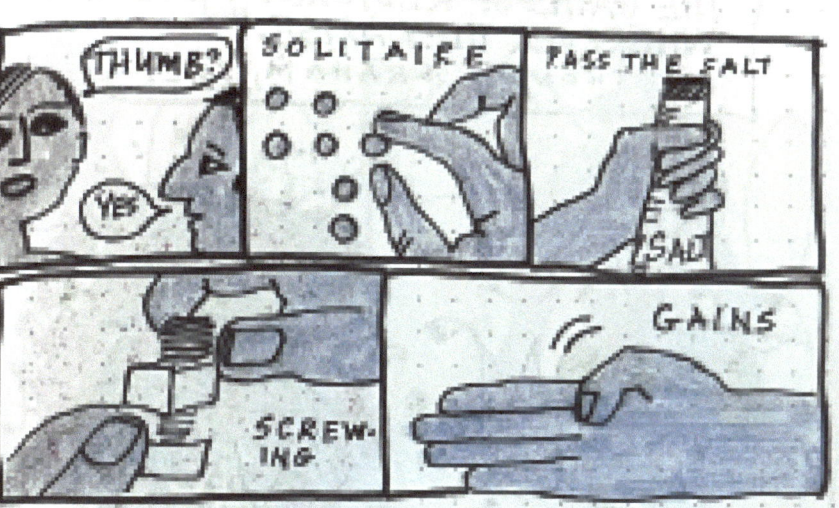

OCCUPATIONAL THERAPY

WEEK 5 IN REHAB AS OUTPATIENT

Thanks to the wonderful therapists at University of Canberra Hospital Rehab Centre, Thomas has regained much mobility in his arm and leg! He's walked 3 kms, lifted 1kg and is comfortable at home and outdoors. The challenge now is to build his strength. Moving up to heavier weights!

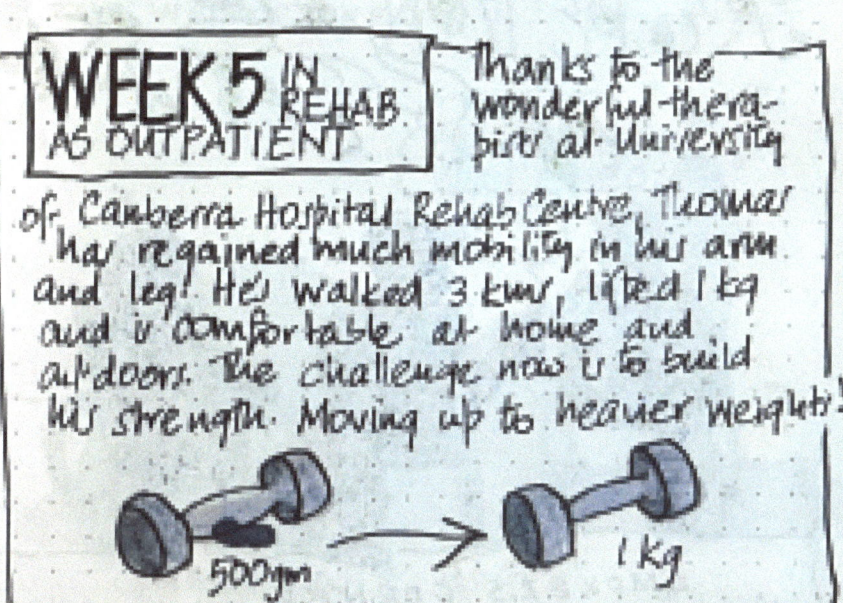

500gm → 1 kg

"STAY FOCUSED. CULTIVATE AN ENGAGED AND POSITIVE MINDSET, AND RECOGNISE AND CELEBRATE THE GAINS OF RESTORED MOVEMENT WHEREVER THEY ARISE."
— THOMAS GRAHAM, JULY 202[?]

THE BLOOM OF REPETITION

SMOKERS CORNER.

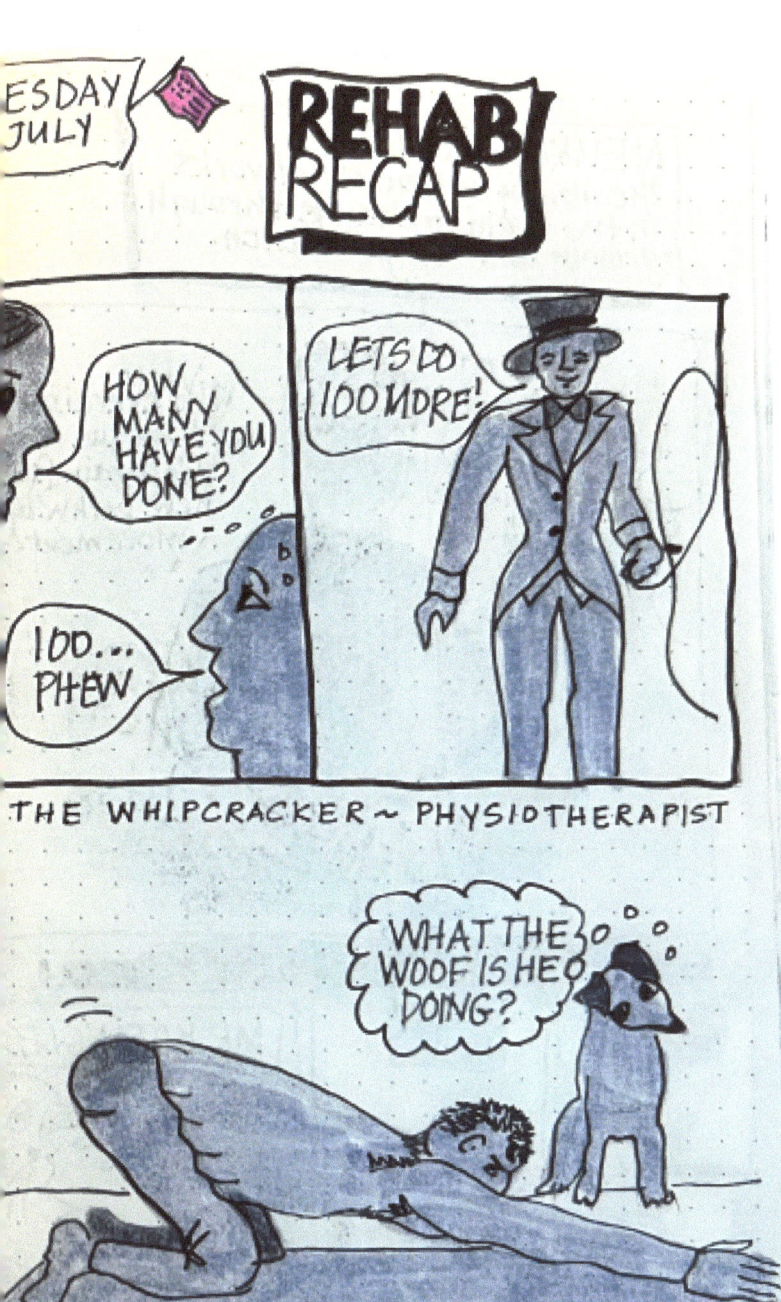

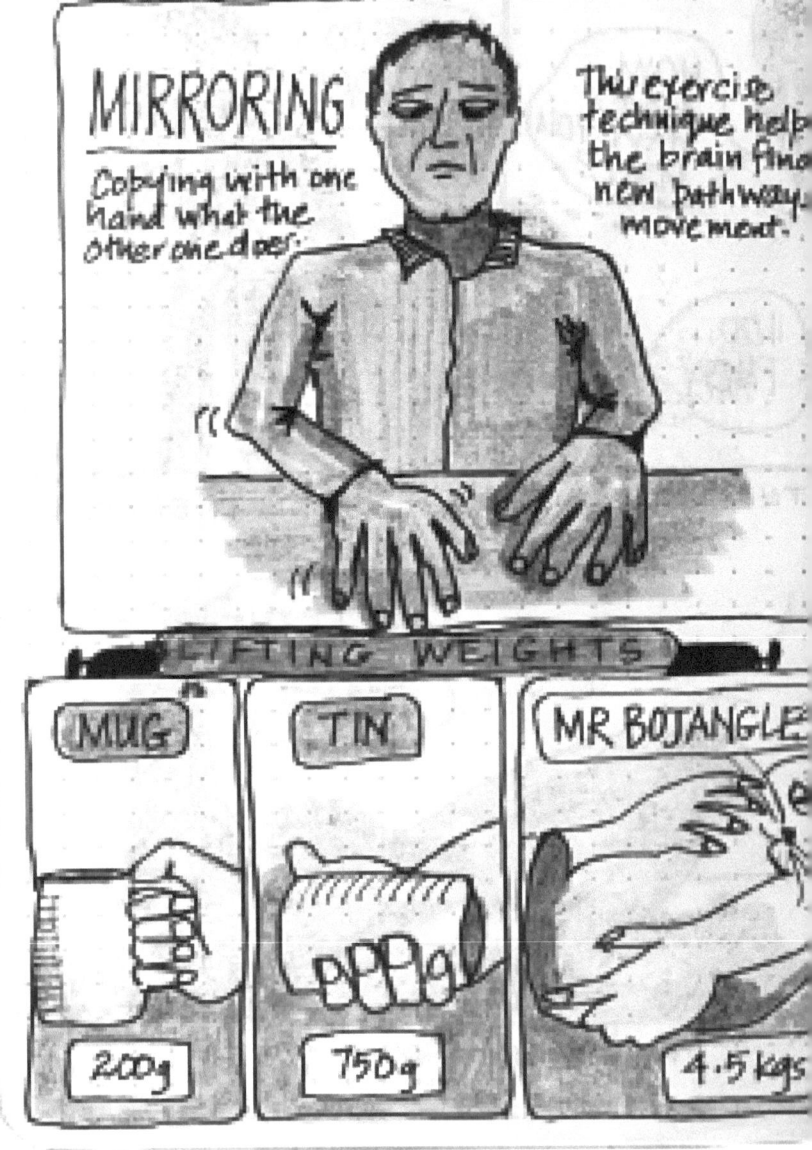

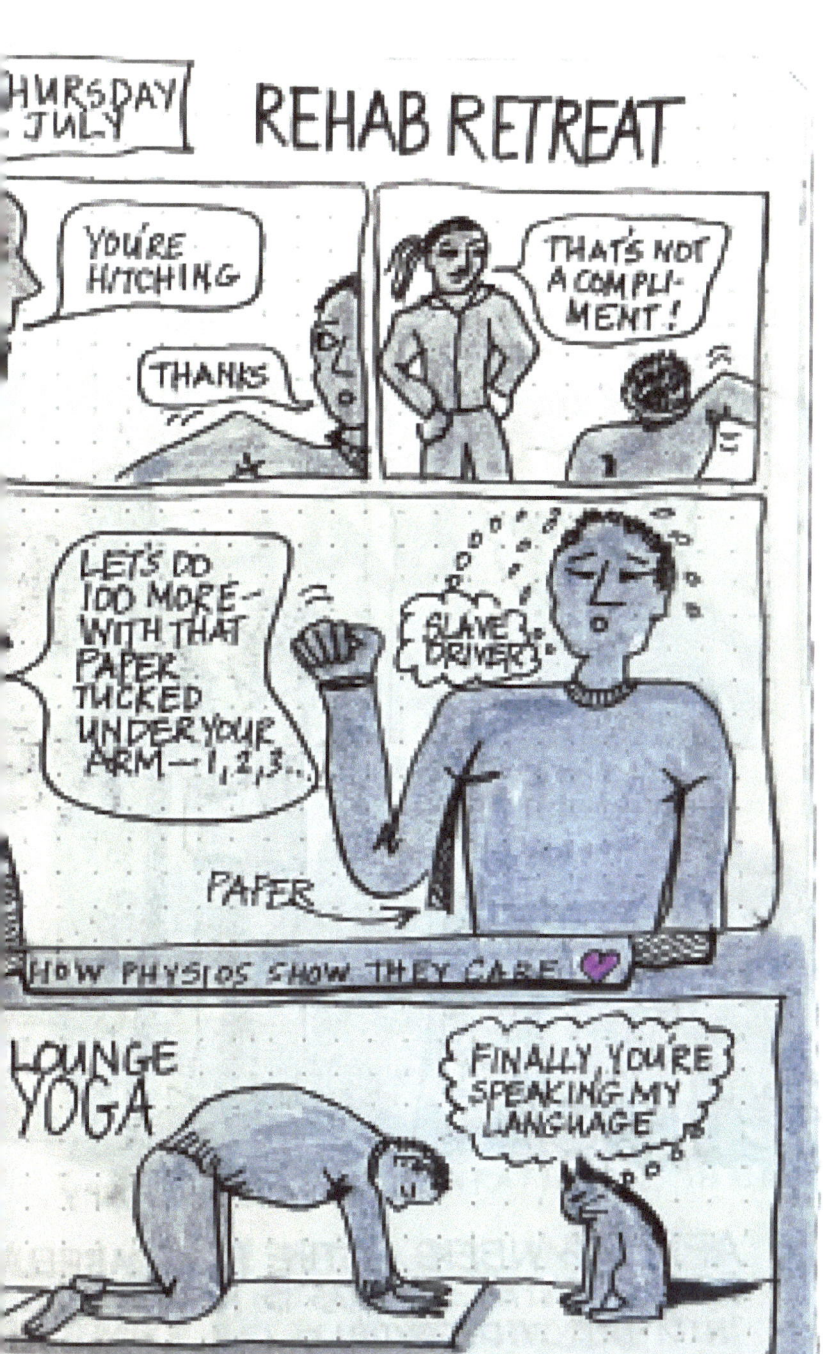

DAY FORTY-THREE

Tuesday, 13 June 2023
Home, Bonner, ACT

Walking backwards into the future

Today it's six weeks since I suffered an ischemic stroke.

Within hours of oxygen ceasing to flow to the left pons region of my brain, I suffered mobility impairment to my limbs on the right side of my body.

Akin to a personal seismic shock, there was no forewarning. In a swift and unexpected twist of fate, my reliable and long-enabled body, faltered.

Suddenly, I faced an uncertain future.

Not being able to stand on my own two feet and walk unaided was confronting, given at one time I'd run a 56km ultramarathon and pre-stroke was capable of hiking 75km over multiple days carrying a 20kg pack. Physical movement is part of my life.

Even more frightening was not being able to lift my right arm, have no movement in my right hand nor use of its fingers. My arm placed in a sling to prevent it from slipping out of its shoulder socket.

The day after the stroke physiotherapist Elyse got me on my feet in front of a mirror and encouraged me to take my first steps. I managed about 20 as she, and her assistant, supported me on either side.

On the same day, Emma, an occupational therapist, wired my forearm to a small device to activate a timed electric charge to simulate my unresponsive hand. Miraculously, my hand opened and closed when the current switched on and off.

Elyse and Emma instilled belief that I could repair my broken body. From the moment they looked me in the eye, they ignited hope that fired an inner resolve. I'm forever grateful for their calm encouragement to embrace self-belief when I wrestled with disbelief.

It was humbling being wired to a heart monitor, my good arm pierced with an intravenous drip, curtailing movement as I was confined to a hospital bed. Even more chastening was nursing assistance to shower—seated in a chair—getting to the toilet or when using a bottle to urinate.

I appreciated being in good hands and care although the setting of an open, acute ward with its harsh artificial lighting, hot air-conditioning and monitoring around the clock, made the days long and challenging, when coupled with the shock of compromised mobility. I certainly missed natural light, fresh air, the outdoors and familiar movement.

I drew comfort from the care, kindness and many good wishes received—from doctors, nurses, therapists, family and friends. The inspiring messages came from everywhere and were significant support for Bobby, who visited me daily and remained steadfast in her equanimity.

Claire, the speech therapist, confirmed that I could swallow normally and retained full speech, both in function and in choosing correct words. In addition, my memory and cognition were unaffected. I could think, discern, imagine and tap into humour, smile and laugh. These retentions were huge—along with the absence of pain—allowing me to focus on restorative thinking, bodily repair and spiritual nourishment.

Apart from the half-hour sessions with Elyse and Emma, I spent short periods standing next to my bed taking my full weight on my legs, shuffling from side to side, doing squats and lifting my right leg up and down. My first basic exercises in five- and ten-minute intervals.

After a week, I was moved to the University of Canberra Rehabilitation Hospital, a short ambulance trip away.

Given my own room and a wheelchair, the facility was modern and spacious, with outdoor courtyards, a large communal gym, dining room and focused physical rehabilitation. Under the care and guidance of a team of therapists—Mel, Emily, Briana, Susanna and Rhein—I spent two weeks in intensive physio exercising four to five hours a day with additional periods in my room, beside or in my bed.

When doing her first assessment, Mel asked me what my goals were.

Three immediately came to mind: I wanted to get home, walk out of the centre independently and feed myself by holding a spoon in my right hand.

I had no idea how long these pivotal functional movements would take to return. I committed myself to whatever the therapists asked me to do.

Physiotherapy is multidimensional. Its aim to restore bodily movement, build strength and regain control over limbs to enable effective function. Its foundation repetitions—endless repeat sets of movement to specific affected parts of the body—shoulder, arm, elbow, forearm, wrist, hand, thumb, fingers and leg, foot and toes.

Primarily, what these physical movements do is teach the brain new neural pathways to activate the movements, naturally.

The brain has the unique capacity to redirect signals to activate these movements to compensate for the loss or damage to the areas of the brain that would normally, and instantaneously, direct such functional movements.

When brain cells in specific locations die during a stroke, it doesn't follow that former movement is lost forever. The brain, when prompted—*I need to move my hand and fingers*—finds another way to activate those movements through the repetitive prompts and repetitious actions to replicate those movements.

This is the marvel of neuroplasticity.

Physiotherapy is the body instructing the brain to respond, the request repeated thousands of times by attempting, and practicing, the actual movement.

Within days of endless repetitions, improvements to my leg allowed me to abandon the wheelchair and walk unaided—my stride ungainly, my balance good, distances short.

When movement and minor strength returned to my shoulder, arm and hand, I removed the sling to begin a new phase of upper body repair—exercising left and right side together in tandem, the affected limbs trying to mimic the smooth, effortless movements of my normal left side.

In addition to being an engaged, active patient with no place for passivity or negative thinking, I practiced other familiar routines, slowly and deliberately, to create a sense of normalcy. Each day I shaved, brushed my teeth, dressed in clean clothes, ate three meals, pitched up at the gym each morning to exercise, showered each evening and relaxed for short periods listening to music on my iPhone.

These small routines along with visits from family and friends, messages of goodwill, the care and kindness of nursing staff, engaging with other stroke survivors with similar drive, and enthusiasm and the daily encouragement and personal challenges set by the therapists, kept my spirits up.

Disappointments and distraction I held at bay—losing my single room when moved to a shared space; a ward and gym lockdown due to a COVID outbreak and a daily blood thinning injection into my abdomen that bloated my tummy and turned the skin black and blue.

My body, fortunately, continued to respond positively to daily exercise.

Small achievements delivered moments of satisfaction—the first time I was able to clasp my two hands firmly together was pure bliss; as was pushing the palms of my hands forward along my naked thighs as I sat on the side of my bed.

Holding a 110ml bottle in my right hand, sufficiently firm, so that I could unscrew the cap and pour milk onto my porridge, a memorable milestone. As was walking independently to the toilet, shower, gym and dining room.

Momentous was using my affected hand to shakingly lift spoonfuls of porridge, upwards and into, my mouth.

All these actions highlighted hope transformed into effective function—the brain/body back working in unison.

After two weeks, I packed my small suitcase and a travel bag with my personal possessions, placed them in the wheelchair and pushed the chair in front of me as I walked out of the rehab facility, bringing an end to 22 days in hospital.

I was going home!

For the past three weeks, I have continued my rehabilitation in the comfort of home with two, weekly, three-hour sessions, at the Brindabella Centre. The outpatient facility and gym at the University of Canberra Hospital under the guidance of a new team of therapists—Kate, Lucy, Tania, Sam and Alex.

Returning home to Bobby, Bojangles and Bibi—wife, pet cat and pet dog—reunited me with family, with all three watchful witnesses to my daily exercises to regain greater movement, more strength and functional control of my affected limbs.

Each morning, I begin with yoga and stretches firmly believing in cultivating uniform balance and movement for my whole body—

my fully enabled left side I want to keep supple, firm and healthy and an example to my right side to regain its full range of subtle movement and greater strength to achieve equilibrium.

Once handrails were installed, the five steps, separating upper and lower levels of the house—initially considered an obstacle of concern—have become part of my exercise course and equipment. Eight metres of lounge carpet together with the steps provide a track for walking and stepping repetitions, with Bojangles and Bibi keeping an eye on every step.

Along with developing greater strength across all limbs, the focus has also been on practices to return the range of finer motor movements—and they are vast in number—to fingertips, thumb control and lifting my arm for above-head movements. Specifically, to hold a pen to write, to fully touch type on my keyboard, to brush my teeth, massage shampoo into my scalp, using my right hand, and to eat with knife and fork. The goal: full function with competent control to mimic natural movement.

These goals are my motivations, tiny achievements to regain mastery of precise movement.

The tactile endpoints to endless repetitive exercises. There is not much fun in counting hundreds of daily repetitions, but there is certainly deeper gratification in the restoration of specific functional movements to achieve activities of daily living.

Physical exercise has changed. When entirely able-bodied, I'd push the limits to get fit and bask in the free flow of endorphins delivering a wave of physiological reward—soothing, energising and filled with a feel-good-factor.

Post-stroke physical exercise is different—sometimes its immediate aftermath is a rushing wave of fatigue. There is certainly deep satisfaction in witnessing the reactivation of basic movement, or when reaching a desired number of controlled repetitions—1, 5, 10, 25, 50 or 100.

More rewarding is knowing once the new neural pathway is established, it sticks—a bit like learning to ride a bicycle, once known, not forgotten. Thereafter, it's about increasing strength, developing greater control, endurance and more speed.

Fatigue comes from the brain/body working out the new pathways to affect movement, the brain burning enormous amounts of energy, as in some areas it's damaged, not unfit.

Learning to pace myself, as well as allowing time to rest, are as important as the exercise itself. Being measured, not impatient in my effort, is key.

After a week at home, I realised I'd been neglecting my right foot as I was focusing exercise on my arm, hand and fingers. My ankle was tight with limited movement to my toes, particularly when wanting to bend them upwards. They didn't respond. This was causing 'drop-foot', my foot tending to drag and angle downwards when walking.

In telling Sam, the physiotherapist, he recommended I practice walking backwards to help with foot flexibility and realignment. I included walking backwards into my daily routines. The results amazing, not only do I have better all-round movement in my ankle and toes, but my gait has also improved to resemble a normal stride, smoothness of step and less of a hitch.

I'm over the moon by the rate and level of recovery since my stroke six weeks ago. I've probably recovered 70% of normal leg and foot movement; 75% of my arm and 90% of hand and finger movements. The remaining percentages lie in finer control which I hope to fully restore in time.

Movement is one scale, strength is another. My leg strength stands at about 70% and arm at 60%—starting from zero, the latter is hugely rewarding and encouraging.

Several months of daily rehab lie ahead as I aim to recover the remaining subtle movement, rebuild strength and stamina within the muscles of the affected limbs. In six weeks, I'll reassess.

My new goals: to drive again, get back into the pool to swim, complete delayed gardening projects, do more recreational activities with Bobby, attempt day long hikes (I've managed a 2.4km walk in an hour with several rest stops), practice idleness and stay healthy.

I'm filled with admiration for the capacity of the body/brain to heal and for the kindnesses and encouragement received from many along the way. These qualities, along with ongoing determination, continued effort and patience, I aim to take with me as I walk backwards into the future to regain full mobility.

DAY FIFTY-FIVE

Sunday, 25 June 2023
Home, Bonner, ACT

Letter in response to Bobby's friend, a long-term yoga teacher

Hi Lynne

Thank you for your kind and insightful response you sent to Bobby last week re my recovery from a stroke.

Initially, your comment suggesting I was a yogi, I found incongruous as I thought if I was a true yogi, I wouldn't have had my stroke in the first place!

Life would be sorted, all the time!

Upon reflection, I'm a likely yogi—trying to fathom the cycles and meaning of life—as I have always done, sometimes with success and sometimes losing my way.

With the recent stroke event, life became more challenging—as one thing I could always rely on—my fully functional enabled body, that defined independent healthy living, is no longer what it was.

It's compromised in several ways—at least temporarily.

The shock of the stroke event and its resultant body impairments has created a different landscape for daily living, one I'm not familiar with.

Restoring motor function, regaining movement, rebuilding strength, remastering control and longer term, reestablishing endurance and speed in the myriad of bodily movements, is not a field I thought I would ever have to play in.

And yet I do. It's here. Now.

Fortunately, I don't have to explain to you—as a restorative lifelong yoga practitioner—repair isn't only about the physicalness of my body—although that remains a primary focus—it's also about mind and spirit; about understanding, meaning and balance as I move through the various phases of recovery.

Almost eight weeks post the event my body is responding well to the daily cycle of physical exercise across upper and lower limbs, their joints, muscles, tendons, ligaments and nerves.

The wonder of neuroplasticity is working. Thank goodness!

Early on, willing an affected hand or foot to move, to lift, to respond to normal function—and it didn't—was very confronting.

With the guidance and benevolent insistence of trained and caring therapists, together with my own intent, determination and effort, the brain/mind has found new pathways to restore function, albeit slowly and from a weak base.

What stands out—as I stood up—is the body's capacity, and seemingly natural inclination, for restoration—knowing that is immensely affirming and gratifying.

Pre-stroke, I looked after my body through regular exercise, healthy eating and avoidance of smoking, excessive alcohol and high stress. Correspondingly, I didn't suffer from high blood pressure or high cholesterol. I was slim and no symptoms of diabetes. Nor do I have issues with my heart, it remains a reliable, safe pump.

My steady road to recovery, I believe, is due to my good health prior to the stroke. If I didn't have that, I would be in a far worse position.

My awareness, alertness and vigilance has been switched on from the beginning. Out of shock and disbelief, and more importantly, in how to affect repair, as my resolve to regain a healthy, functioning physicalness remains, despite the assault on my brain and some impairment.

You write of an *'unchanging witness throughout'*. About twenty years ago, I was introduced and became aware of the *'observing self'*, that part of ourselves that is able to watch, be aware and witness awareness, beyond the thinking and physical self.

The discovery was revelatory and over the years I've continued to maintain this awareness through meditation (being here now practice, through Pilates and walking) and completing several *Acceptance and Commitment Therapy (ACT)* courses with Dr Russ Harris, medical practitioner and author of several books, including *The Reality Slap*.

I'm assuming your reference to the *'unchanging witness throughout'* is akin, if not a close equivalent, to/of the *'observing self'* which I'm mindful of in my recovery, both in regaining physical movement, in all its subtle forms, and in the mental capacity, to stay engaged and positive.

At the beginning of most days, I do stretches and yoga exercises to bring balance and free flowing movement to my body, believing physical wellness is holistic, involving the whole body, not just about restoring the damaged bits. These exercises bring equilibrium to all parts, in contrast to the physiotherapy, which focuses exclusively on the limbs, joints and muscles requiring direct, intensive repair.

The mindfulness, stretching and yoga movements complement the physiotherapy, in fact they're vital, bringing a more complete restoration, as the impaired limbs learn from the enabled limbs. For me, it's also about the sensation and joy of movement, not just about the mechanics.

I've entered a new phase of recovery, as much physical as it is psychological—thankfully, most movement has returned to the affected limbs. They are, however, still weak, endurance is low and speed reduced. Its going to take several months to rebuild greater strength—a lot of repetitions.

Maintaining a sustained programme of steady exercise is key, as is accepting a slower pace and gradual progress. I tend to be impatient. Being *patient* consistently, needs to become a new behaviour, working in tandem with the physical exercises.

Easier thought than done!

In the coming weeks, I'm seeking to develop a calmness—open and aware to accepting I have time for the body/brain to heal—to rebuild strength and for the mind/spirit to be patient as I adjust to changes in my body's capacity and a different tempo to daily living.

A work in progress for head, body and heart . . .

Regards
Thomas

DAY SIXTY-THREE

Monday, 3 July 2023
Home, Bonner, ACT

Letter in response to a friend living in South Africa

Hi Graham

Sorry to hear you suffered an ischemic stroke that has affected mobility to the left side of your body, with current impairment to your left hand.

Experiencing a stroke is a confronting experience. It causes shock, disbelief.

The stroke severity and location within the brain differs from person to person, as does an individual's rate and response to recovery.

You received emergency care early, including clot-busting medication, you've started occupational therapy and physiotherapy and have restored function and movement to some areas that were first affected.

That is all good news.

I fully understand the confronting nature of lost functional movement. I experienced that myself in the first weeks post-stroke and have since been steadily regaining movement, control and strength to my affected right arm and leg.

My whole right arm, hand and fingers were limp and non-responsive with my arm held in a sling to ensure the shoulder didn't slip from its socket.

It was my dominant limb too, so I needed to do everything with my non-dominant arm and hand, including typing with one finger on my iPhone (I have since returned to full touch typing, albeit slowly).

What helped me was embracing belief in neuroplasticity while focusing on consistent exercise of the affected limbs.

You'd know the drill—countless repetitions.

What I've learnt in my own recovery (two months in) is that the journey is part physical, mental and spiritual. You need to work on all three.

It's been scientifically and medically proven that the brain can re-organise itself to bring movement back to affected limbs when the area, usually controlling this movement in the brain, is damaged—when it literally dies.

Read about neuroplasticity, believe it and embrace it. This is part of the mental component I believe is essential for recovery.

The Brain That Changes Itself, by Norman Doidge, is worth reading.

Physically, Mel, my OT, wired my affected arm to a FES (Functional Electronic Stimulation) device, for 30-minute sessions, to get my limp hand to open and close (which it did).

In time, a glass bottle (standard herb container) was placed in the hand which I tried to clasp each time the programmed electrical charge opened my hand, and when the charge switched off, closed it.

I worked off that, starting with the slightest twitch of movement without the device, to believe, will and imagine my fingers and hand moving.

I also did a lot of exercise on my wrist—repetitions of raising my wrist when placed on a rolled towel. I could barely raise it to begin with but kept trying—even if there was only a hint of movement.

In recovery, you keep trying and don't give up!

Also, keep in mind that your hand is attached to your arm. Exercising and strengthening the network of muscles in your forearm and upper arm will facilitate hand movement. I used a yellow theraband (big elastic band, resistance graded to a colour code) tied to the side of my hospital bed to exercise arm muscles while lying in bed.

Think it. Believe it. Exercise it. Repeatedly and rest. Rest is very important, as the muscles require periods of relaxation as much as they do exertion.

The occupational therapists and physiotherapists primary focus is on recovery of functional movement. That is their role. Listen to what they say, advise and practice.

Be an active participant in your recovery. Give them feedback and experiment. If something isn't working after repetitive practice—modify, tweak or change.

My experience is that they are creative and encouraging—they're open to try new things.

Their focus is on repair of affected limbs. I look at my whole body as a unit. I believe in balance and free flowing movement within my whole body.

The working limbs can teach the affected limbs. Get your left hand to mimic the movement of your right hand. Watch the two of them working together. Imagine them working together.

Use your right hand to massage the fingers and palm of your left hand while you sit watching TV or before going to bed or whenever you can do so.

Doing your own exercises outside of the formal rehab sessions is important to facilitate recovery.

I do a lot of stretching and yoga exercises for my whole body—do not neglect the rest of your body while attending to your left hand and arm.

Exercise to keep the whole body supple, strong and striving for free flow of natural movement.

Normal functional limbs can remind the affected areas what natural movement is and instruct your brain to find new pathways to restore movement to all areas.

Be patient—I'm impatient, so patience is a new learning for me!

The journey can be slow—accept that—it's as psychological and spiritual as it is physical. Over time, develop practices in all three domains for effective recovery.

Stay focused, cultivate an engaged and positive mindset, and recognise and celebrate the gains of restored movement, wherever they arise.

All the best
Thomas

(Note: It was most gratifying when Graham, who has a sister living in Sydney, flew from South Africa to Australia to visit her, and drove to Canberra, to see Bobby and I several months after our correspondence).

DAY SIXTY-SIX

Thursday, 6 July 2023
Home, Bonner, ACT

'Brindy' rehab

Today ends my formal post-stroke rehabilitation at the Brindabella Day Centre. The bi-weekly sessions, over six weeks, have flown by.

I began intensive rehab three weeks after being struck by an ischemic stroke that affected my mobility and movement to my right side and limbs.

On Tuesday and Thursday mornings, Bobby has driven me to 'Brindy', to watch the first 10 minutes of my rehab, then retreat to the café for a coffee and to sketch—her mindful practice to manage her changed world, pausing much of her own life, to be a carer and supportive companion of mine.

I walked in for the first appointment with a weak leg, staggered gait, and floppy foot—that angled downwards—the toes unable to move up or down. Ungainly, a likely self-activating trip hazard! Similarly, my arm and hand—which had recently regained their functional movement—were weak, lacked finer motor control and had limited power and endurance.

I couldn't grasp comfortably or keep firm control of movement, my right thumb a reticent communicator with its neighbouring fingers. Picking up a glass to drink, holding my toothbrush, peeling a potato, touch typing or using a knife and fork, all beyond me.

My right shoulder, arm and wrist were mobile, yet equally weak—a few pushes of a vacuum cleaner exhausting, as was one or two repetitions wiping a tabletop; ditto my inability to lift my arm above my shoulder to shampoo my hair while showering; or trying to glide the electric razor across my face when shaving; or attempting to remove a cup from the kitchen cupboard when making tea for Bobby and I.

Driving was prohibited, gardening halted, lengthy outdoor walks paused and swimming aspirational. These limitations appear small, yet big in the context of convenient, able-bodied daily living.

With the guidance and benevolent instruction of Kate, Tania, Sam and Alex—my team of occupational therapists and physiotherapists—I set to work following their exercise programmes, in two and a half hour sessions, to revive mastery of movement and to build strength and endurance.

I've remained focused, cultivating an engaged and positive mindset to sustain motivation. And to recognise and celebrate the gains of controlled movement, wherever these arise. The body has responded well to the challenges set—sufficient to stimulate and achieve targets, yet not to cause pain (discomfort is acceptable).

Occasionally, I'd push a little too hard to be greeted with fatigue. It hits like a giant wave, its suddenness disturbing, though fleeting—not to cause alarm, just an awareness of a new body experience to manage and let pass.

Daily, I repeated many of the exercises at home, along with yoga, stretches and active mental stimulation—through reading and courses—to learn the wonders of neuroplasticity and nurture resilience to navigate life's pathways post-stroke.

After each rehab session, Bobby and I catch up with Bill—a fellow stroke survivor who continues his rehabilitation in the University of Canberra Hospital, alongside 'Brindy'.

Bill and I met during my time in the hospital and forged a friendship in adversity. Each evening we chat on the phone to inspire each other, reflect on progress or hiccups, and to laugh.

Yesterday, he excitedly told me he could return home for the first time in three months, to continue his recovery at HOME, with Patricia, his partner, and Benji, his cat, in regional NSW. Great news.

After six weeks of rehab my walking is near to natural again—my foot and ankle back to normal (thanks to backward walking). I can wiggle my toes!

I'm regularly walking 2km in a single stretch—slow and steady with Bibi, our pet dog. Whoopie!

I can touch-type again, massage my head with my right palm, use a knife and fork, peel potatoes for dinner, cook dinner and hold a glass comfortably to drink refreshing water. Shoulder hitches are becoming less and less.

I still have to build more muscle strength for endurance in both my arm and leg—this will come with independent, ongoing exercise in the months ahead. Driving, swimming and hiking await.

I'm learning to be patient, recognising this is about acceptance and tolerance of life's rhythms—not a reference to someone needing medical treatment!

My ongoing recovery could not have been done without Bobby and my team of therapists. To Kate, Tania, Sam and Alex, a big THANK YOU.

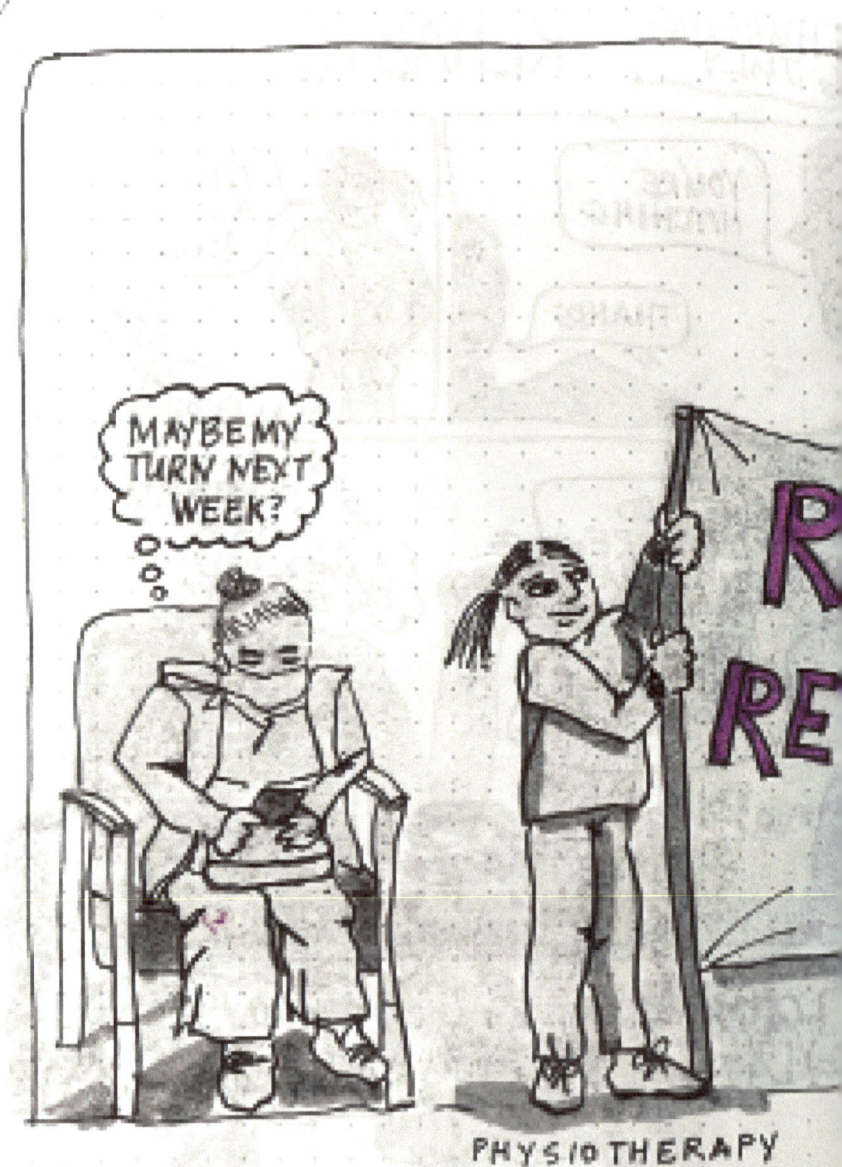

ESDAY JULY

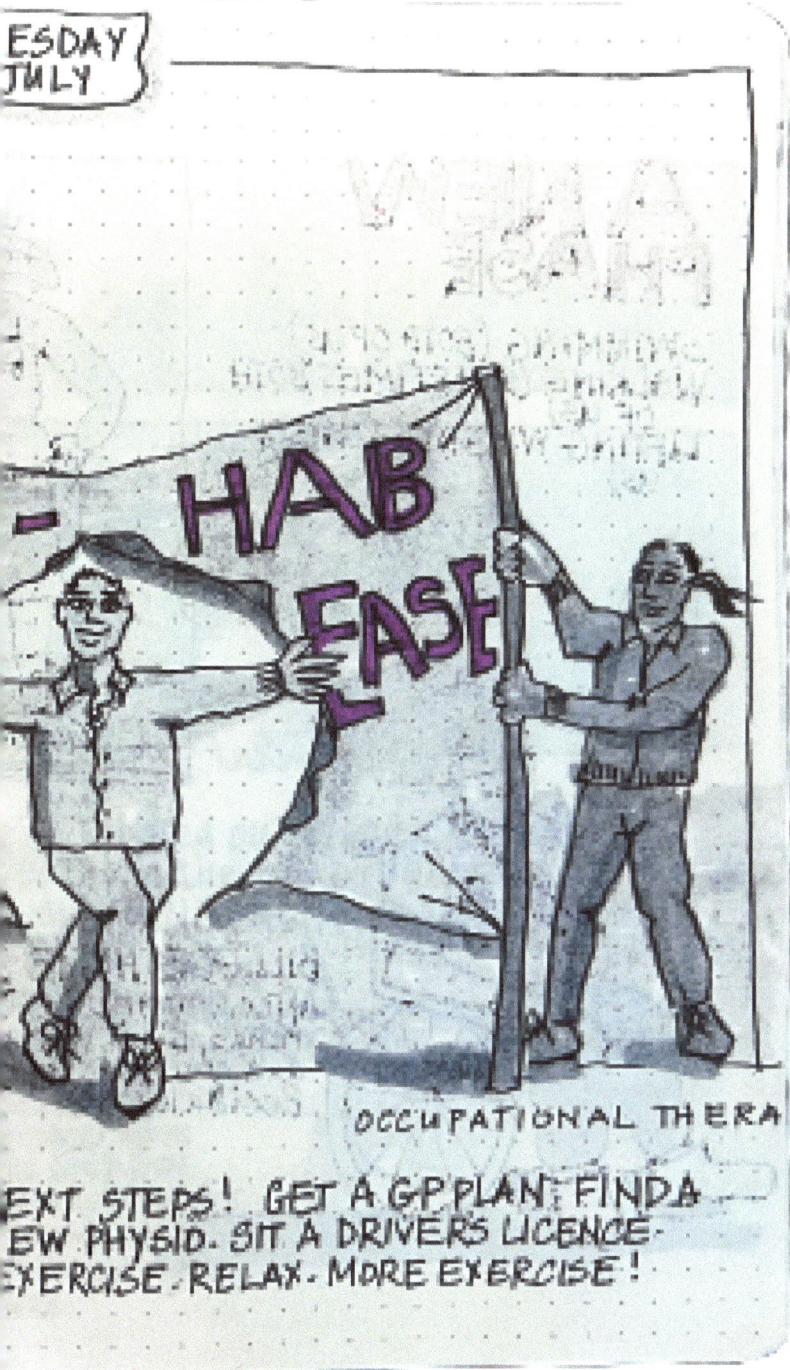

OCCUPATIONAL THERA

EXT STEPS! GET A GP PLAN. FIND A
EW PHYSIO. SIT A DRIVERS LICENCE.
EXERCISE. RELAX. MORE EXERCISE!

A NEW PHASE

SWIMMING (BOTH OF US)
WALKING (SOMETIMES BOTH OF US)
LIFTING WEIGHTS (ONE OF US)

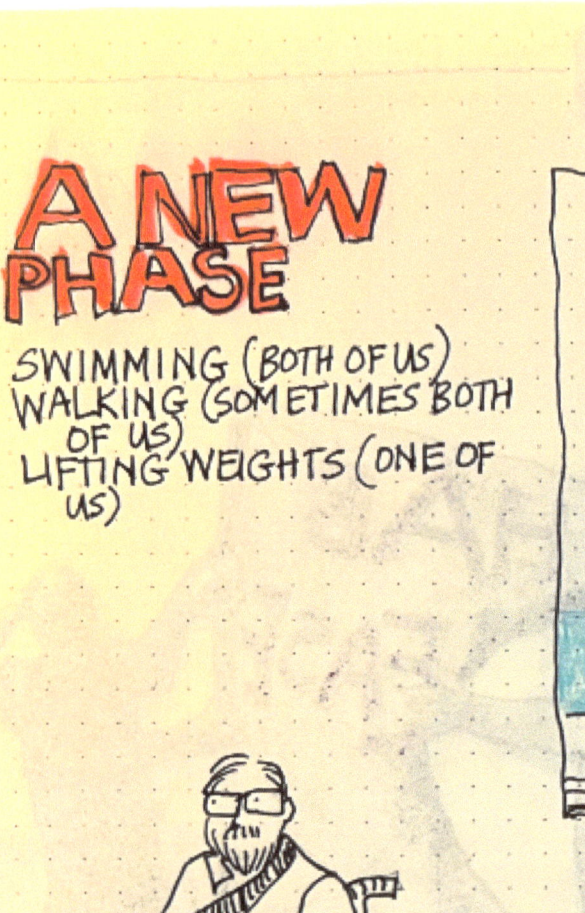

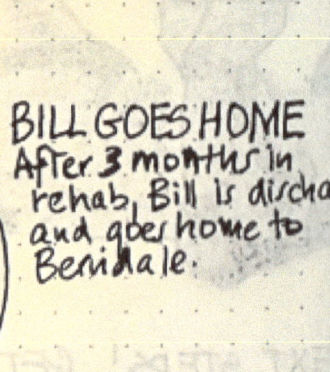

BILL GOES HOME
After 3 months in rehab, Bill is discharged and goes home to Benidale.

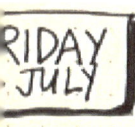

SWIM THERAPY

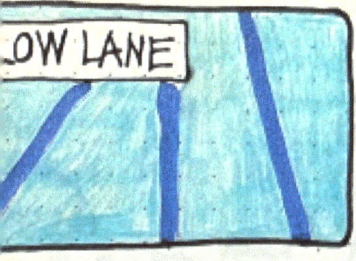

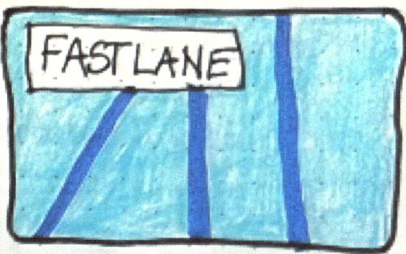

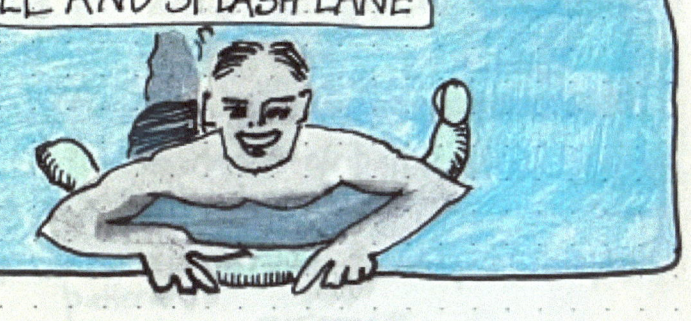

We've replaced outpatients' rehab therapy with swim therapy on Tuesday and Thursday at the GUNGHALIN LEISURE CENTRE.

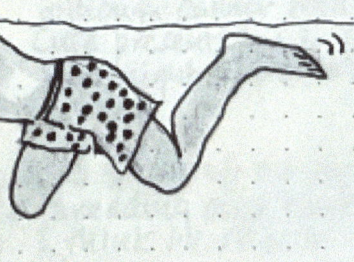

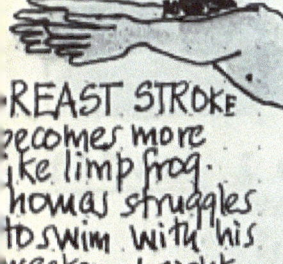

BREAST STROKE becomes more like limp frog. Thomas struggles to swim with his weakened right side.

TUESDAY 19 JULY — **TUESDAY THERAPY**

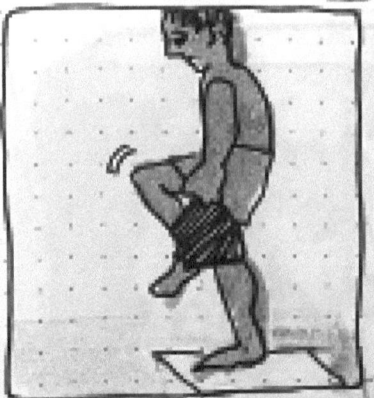
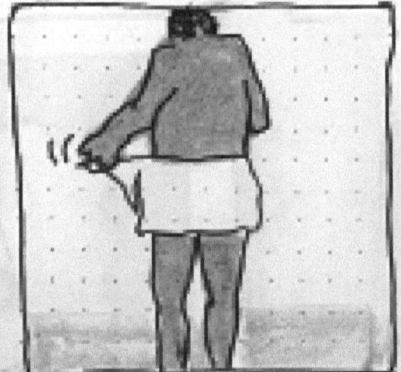

THE SWIMMING POOL SHUFFLE

Getting dressed as a stroke survivor can be challenging. Pulling on and pulling off bathers at the baths is particularly tricky. We rewarded ourselves with coffee and banana cake at the WILD BARK visitor centre at Mulligans Flat.

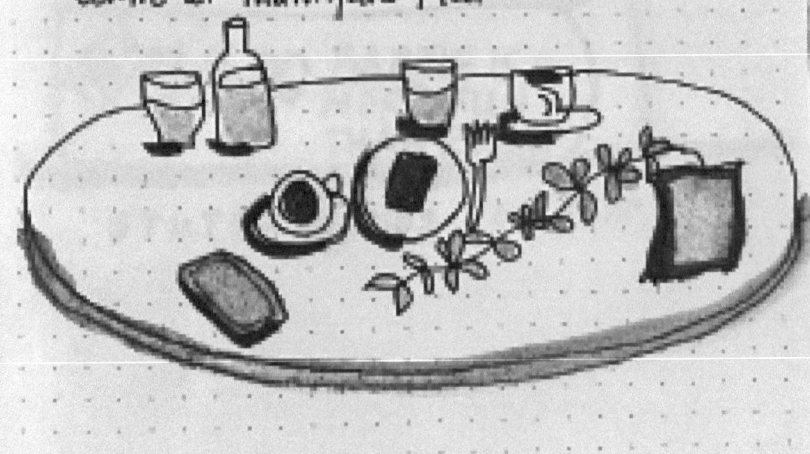

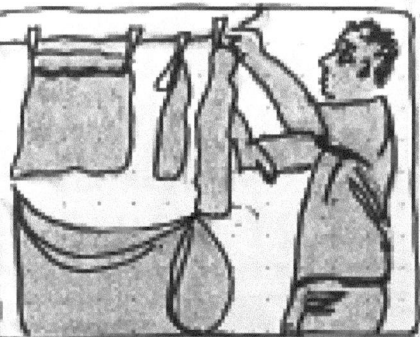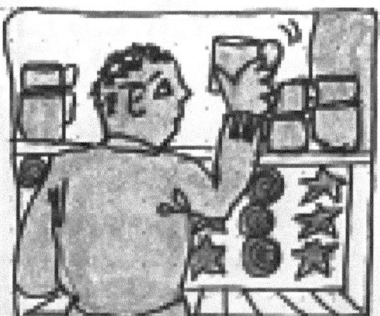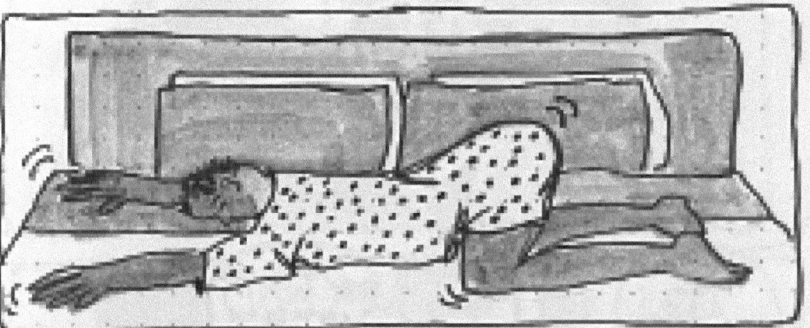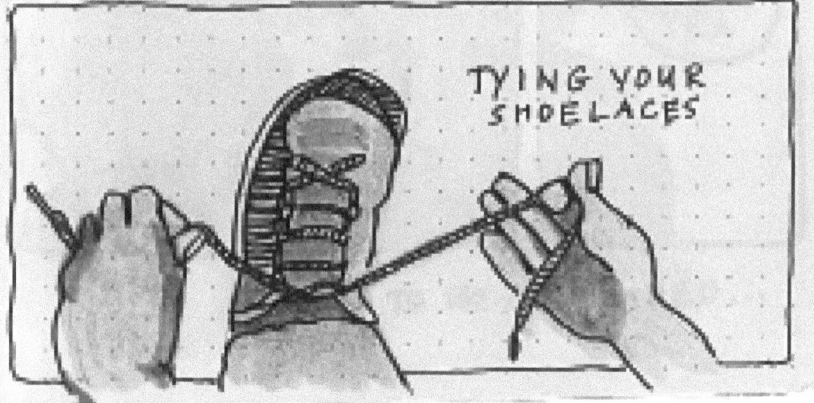

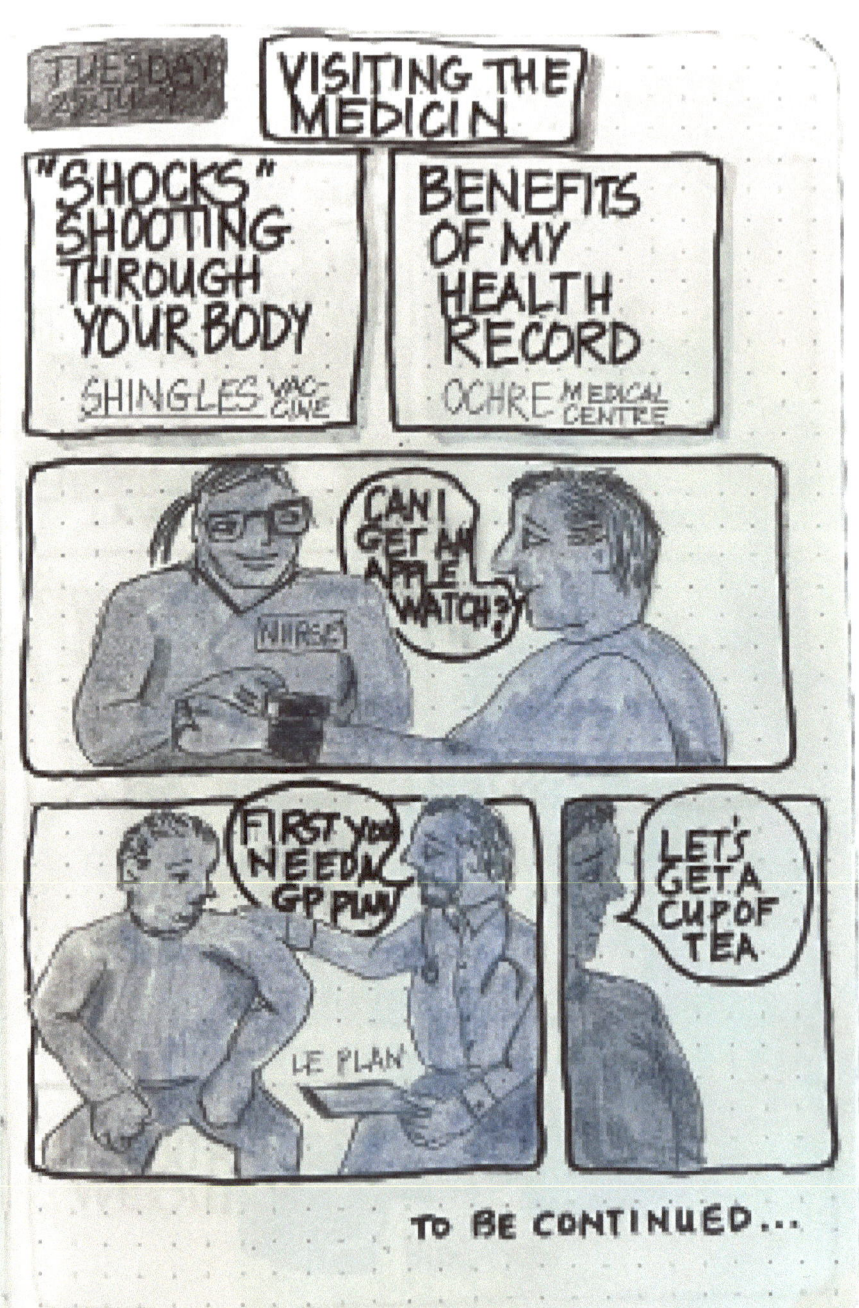

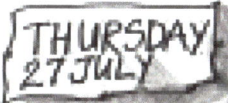

MOMENTUM MAGIC

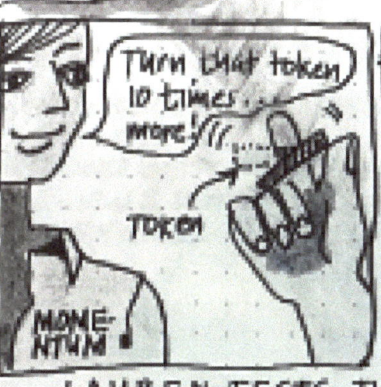
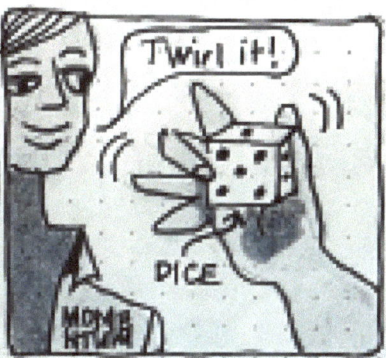

LAUREN TESTS THOMAS'S FINGERTIPS.

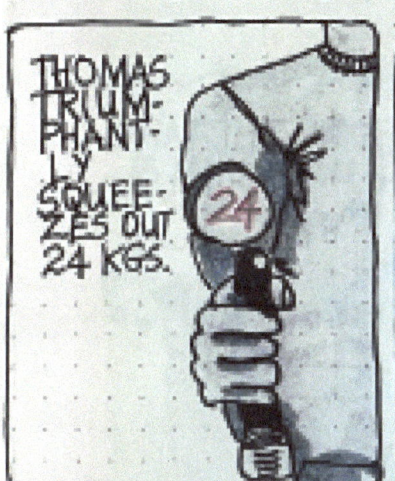
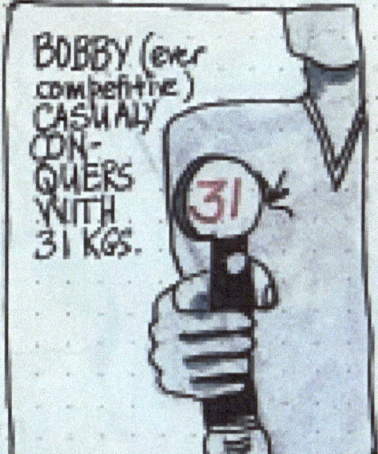

TESTING OUR HAND GRIP STRENGTH

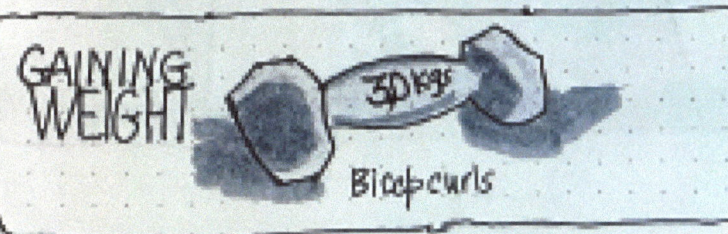

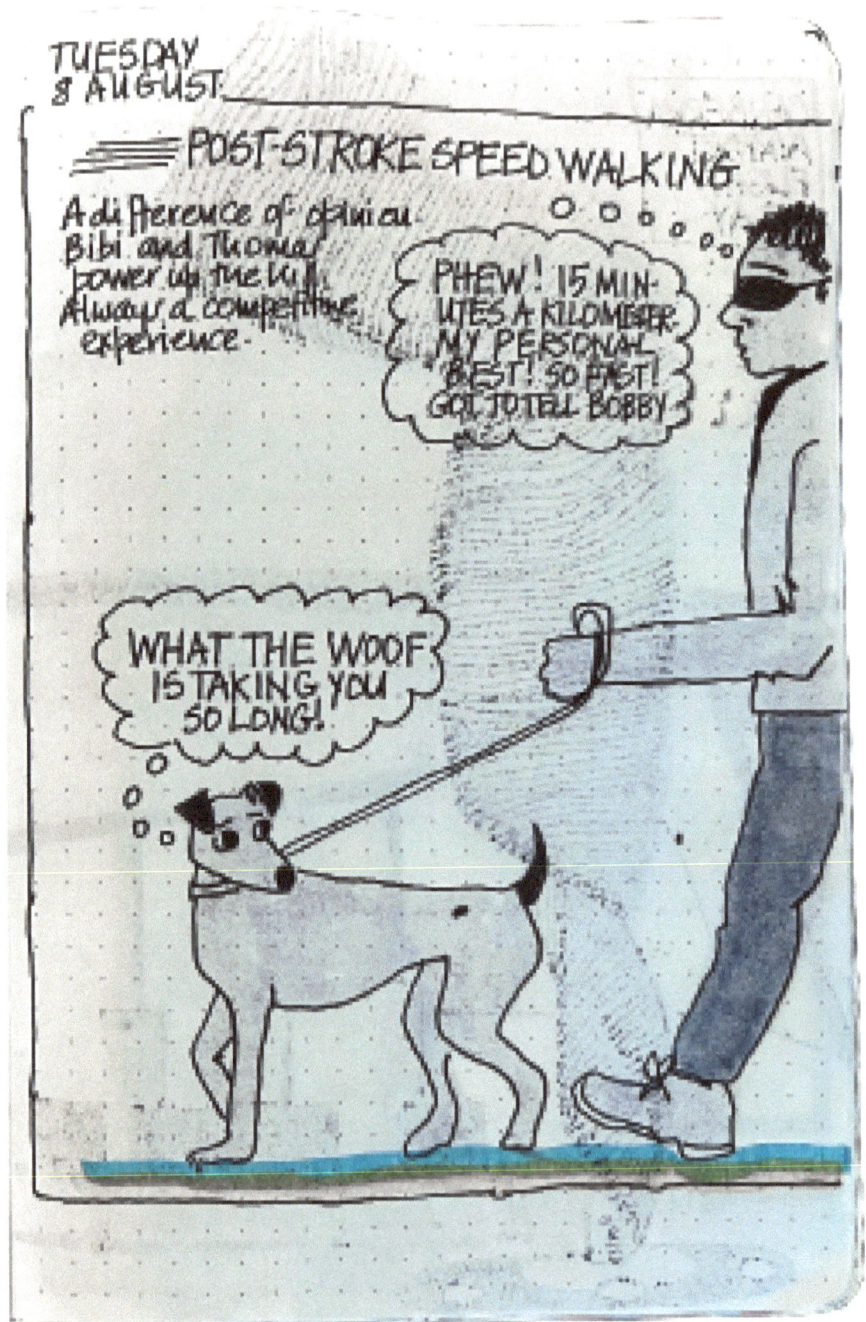

DAY EIGHTY-FIVE

Tuesday, 25 July 2023
Home, Bonner, ACT

Three Months

Three months since struck by stroke
deep shock embedded with disbelief

Functional movement lost on right side
suspending able-bodiedness

Impaired mobility—for how long?
Real fear reflected in limp limbs

Belief, body and brain bridge neural pathways
Learning to move again, slowly

Intensive exercise, repeated again and again
Building strength, stamina, adept coordination

Companionship—Bobby escorting, driving, sharing breakfast,
lunch and supper, watching Sarah Ferguson on the 7.30 Report

*Joy—wiggling toes, clasping hands, cupping palms, carpet yoga
drifting into soothing sleep, awakening to sunlit frosty mornings*

*Satisfaction—walking Bibi to Golden Sun Moth Hill
casting eyes across Canberra to the Brindabellas*

*Delight—holding a knife and fork, tying shoelaces, cuddling Bojangles
opening a rip top can, touch typing—mastering finer motor skills*

*Three months post-stroke I smile, give thanks, for all the support
Lost movement restored, wellness returning, life on course once more.*

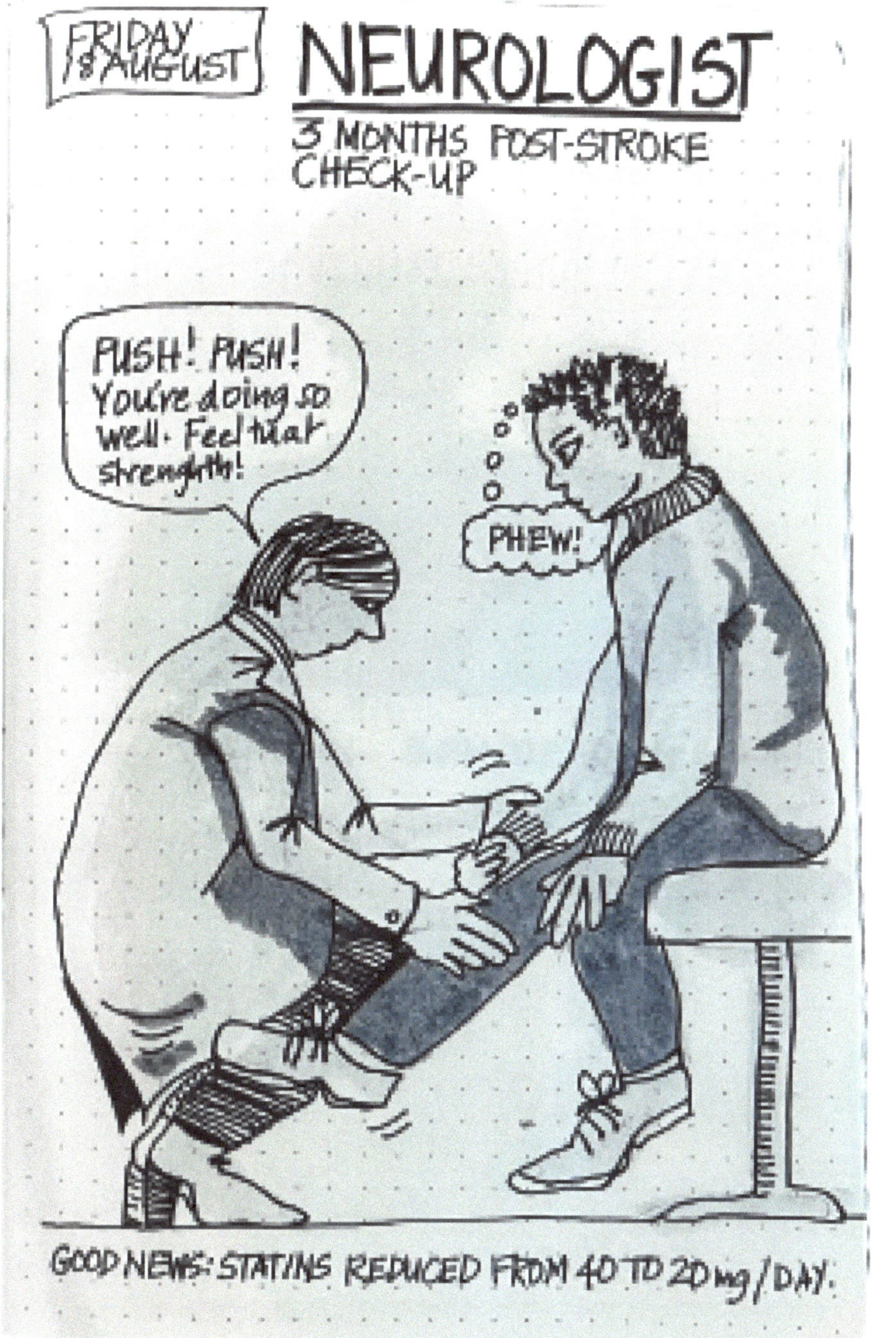

DAY ONE HUNDRED AND EIGHTY-FIVE

Thursday, 2 November 2023

Home, Bonner, ACT

Entering the age of senescence

It's six months since I was struck by a stroke. The assault momentarily starved blood and oxygen to a spot in my brain, causing a cluster of cells to die, resulting in a period of paralysis to my right-sided limbs.

I've been in recovery since, restoring movement and strength to affected limbs to enable independent living.

I prefer *restoration* to *recovery* as a descriptor, as post severe stroke there is seldom full recovery. Not all functions return immediately, or completely, and some remain weak, lingering as works in progress, requiring further rehabilitation.

Restoring function to limp limbs and weak muscles, as well as rebuilding their strength and stamina, is a slow process. It requires deliberate, daily exercise, diligently done, with patience.

These are some of my learnings of recent months.

Restoration requires both brain and body to work in unison.

This is typical of general life function but the critical point of difference—post-stroke—is the brain has to establish new neural pathways to reinstate normal function to affected limbs. The brain cells previously controlling this function, are no longer active, they're dead.

Endless repetitions of physical movement remind the brain the affected limb function *is* still required, calling on other cells to step in, to provide the impulses for normal function. In sporting terms, it's going to the bench to bring on reserves for injured players who cannot continue.

My neuroplastic brain is actively engaged in cell rewiring and strengthening to restore function to affected limbs—doing so silently, outside of consciousness and without brain pain. And it's made good progress.

In contrast—and in tandem—my body has had to do the heavy lifting, completing thousands of physical repetitions to get my right arm and leg to lift, fingers to grasp and clasp, ankle to flex and toes to wiggle, to restore mobility. At the most basic level, so I can feed and clean myself, and walk.

Unlike brain rewiring, restoring limb and muscle function, is conscious, visible and tactile.

Although I've succeeded in restoring primary function to my affected limbs, the muscles are not retaining their strength as readily as they did when doing fitness training pre-stroke. They're getting stronger, show improvements to endurance, but do so slowly and incrementally, as the newly established neural pathways, themselves need to build impulse speed and strength. By analogy, it's as if my arm and leg muscles require 100 volts for normal function but the newly formed circuits are only providing 75 volts. Calling on the brain to deliver more voltage is a work in progress, as I'm learning.

In this restoration phase, I'm slower and weaker than I used to be. I'm adjusting to senescence—facing up to a deteriorating body, marked through ageing and a slap to my brain.

I think, therefore, I am what I used to be. In reality, I'm not.

I think I'm my former self; my slower/weaker body, however, reminds me I'm not, as my post assault brain, as the primary control centre, is itself having to find new ways to deliver functional performance to my reviving limbs.

It's a weird state to be in—brain *and* body repair—the one silent and invisible and the other filled with sweat, toil, grunts and niggles.

Hurrying is what I used to be, as pre-stroke I was always in command and coordinated, with no impediments to doing physical tasks quickly, easily and to completion. I was blessed with high energy, dexterity, practical acumen, aided by complete able-bodiedness.

In over sixty years, I never saw my body having any fault lines— and then wham, out of the blue, came the brain assault.

I'm not unusual as strokes strike many around the world each year. A quick Google search gives the annual global number as 15 million, as reported by the World Health Organisation. A third die, a third are left permanently disabled and the remainder learn to deal with degrees of lighter impairment as best as they can.

Closer to home, a wall poster at my local medical centre signals: *One Australian has a heart attack or stroke every four minutes,* reinforcing the prevalence of cardiovascular disease. In the USA, its one American every 40 seconds.

I count myself lucky as I retained my speech, cognition, memory and core movement, though initially lopsided. Post-stroke and formal rehabilitation, I'm left with debilities, characterised by muscle weakness, rather than disability. I'm able, independently, to engage in most activities of daily living, overcoming the temporary paralysis to my right side, through intensive exercise.

Dealing with the effects of stroke go beyond the physical assault on brain and body function.

Mentally, during the first 48 hours post-stroke, I was equally struck by shock and disbelief—what had happened, to me? Why now? What next?

I wept at my loss of limb function when looking at my rigid right leg and foot, frozen hand and limp arm, the latter supported in a sling. The thought of permanent disability, a frightening possibility and unwelcome bedfellow.

The tears were important, releasing stressful tension, rather than expressions of self-pity. Their flow sourced an inner strength, igniting a fierce determination to set out and discover what function I could restore to my affected limbs? That became my daily priority in the weeks and months ahead.

Mental fortitude and spiritual comfort become close allies after suffering a stroke. Without them, it's difficult to sustain the constant discipline of physical effort when endeavouring to regain limb function, to enable mobility. I reminded myself that decades before I'd trained to run an ultramarathon, over many months. I imagined regaining my mobility would be akin to training again for a gruelling, long race. I'd done it before—twice—so I could do it again. I had the time, I just needed to focus on effort. And I did.

I'm not suggesting mental resilience can only come from a physical challenge. Adversity comes in many forms as does finding sources for calm, courage and commitment to get through low points, from pure survival to thriving wellness. Embracing these vital qualities is important to supplement spiritual sustenance, whatever the personal preference. Be it meditation, prayer, yoga, self-reflection, creative pastimes, and, additionally, for me, gardening and slow walks along local paths, witnessing the falling leaves of autumn and, with passing seasons, admiring the new growth of spring.

Equally important during physical restoration are social supports—people—to help, inform, comfort and inspire along the way. I've been enriched by kindness and the assistance I've received from many during my rehabilitation, whether from the medical and health profession, close family and friends—near and far—casual acquaintances, or when crossing paths with fellow stroke survivors. These encounters have kept my spirits up and the menace of depression at bay.

My body has responded well to its rehab program as I progressed from acute care, into rehab hospital, then to out-of-home physio care, before landing currently, at do-it-yourself-care. Through these phases, I've maintained motivation and commitment to exercising without becoming captive to the process, making sure to prune the roses—over three slow sessions—and enjoy the scent of first blooms that currently fill my garden.

There have been some testing times and challenges.

Losing Bojangles, my pet cat of 16 years, three months post-stroke, was akin to another body blow. It hurt and saddened me. Bo was a daily constant companion, a loyal friend, the inspiration for my small business, Mr Petman, and a great comfort once returning home from hospital. When writing, he always lay close to me. His loss is deeply felt as a valuable, now missing, member of the family.

The most annoying, niggling post-stroke disruptor has been statin body wars.

Statin medication is one of the world's most prescribed medications for cardiovascular disease, including stroke survivors. It's designed to reduce the production of cholesterol—principally LDL cholesterol, often referred to as 'bad' cholesterol, as the sticky fat-like substance, which the body readily produces in abundance as part of normal life function. LDL has the potential to narrow arteries by coating them with plaque that can impede blood flow. This, along with blood clot formation, can block vital blood and oxygen to the brain, causing life-threatening strokes.

Once a stroke survivor—regardless of other risk factors—the medical profession sees LDL cholesterol as a potential hazard to control and, statins, sold under many brand names, is the medication of first choice, to minimise the repetition of having another stroke event.

Statins, I discovered—at least the brand I'm prescribed—have negative side-effects for muscles. They ache, stiffen and become sore, 24/7 (this is my experience, others may have an entirely different, possibly neutral reaction).

Three months in, despite restoring primary functional movement and muscle strength to my affected limbs, I felt awful. My muscles, regardless of time of day, whether I exercised or rested them, ached incessantly. All movement became uneasy, making me grumpy and morose (confirmed by Bobby). The impact bilateral, even my good muscles on my unaffected left side, would stiffen and ache.

These side-effects took the shine off all that was positive about getting well again. It felt like a paradoxical regression—overall my mobility, strength and general wellness was improving, yet my muscles screamed in protest, they hurt. At my three months check in with Dr Sales, my neurologist, she agreed to halve the dose to see whether this would ease the discomfort.

Another month went by without relief, so I decided, independently, to take a statin holiday. The results, amazing. Within three days I felt relief, and within five, was my old self, movement free flowing, the absence of pain and discomfort invigorating.

After a week, I returned to the medication at an even lower dose, continuing to seek quality statin intolerance data online and by asking friends and acquaintances whether they took the medication—even my neighbour didn't escape! I was surprised just how many took statins, more for cardio than stroke.

I built an informal medicine chest of comparative info about statin brands, doses and impacts. I also followed medical advice and spoke to my GP about my negative reaction to the medication. A Frenchman, and avid rugby union supporter, I first had to discuss rugby wars, extending him an olive branch for the Springboks knocking out the Tricolours, a few weeks before, at the Rugby World Cup in Paris.

Getting down to a statin scrummage, he was adamant I had to stay on the medication, and we mutually agreed on a dosage before another blood test in three months. I'm hoping it will match my previous cholesterol test results—at the four-month mark—which were exemplary, as is my blood pressure. If my muscles continue to rebel, he'll prescribe a different brand.

Throughout the six months, Bobby has documented our post-stroke journey, with daily sketches in a visual journal. Witnessing a life-threatening event, and its aftermath, is hardest on those that are closest. Partners feel the impact emotionally and practically as they become the spine in support of physical restoration and framing new normalcy. Having to be strong and supportive, under the weight of uncertainty and upheaval to routines, is huge.

As much as I needed support, so did Bobby, in areas I've already touched on—emotionally, spiritually and socially. Thankfully, family, friends and colleagues stepped up, and in, to help her—most notably, Louis, our son. Collectively, these kind actions were, and are, deeply appreciated, by both of us.

By nature, Bobby is a networker, explorer and pragmatic—steeled with equanimity. In solitary, quiet moments she turned to Bibi—her pet fox terrier—and to her art—journaling, sketching, drawing, painting and tutoring—to strengthen her equanimous leanings. These provided lightness, companionship and a restorative attention focus, while I took the first steps to get back on my feet and a myriad of exercises, to restore functionality to my arm, hand and fingers.

Recently, Bobby produced an artwork of me—*Post Stroke Blues*—which last week won first prize at the annual exhibition of the Artists Society of Canberra, in the Digital Art category. Selling on the first day, too. A just reward and recognition for her marathon, as a close-up support person.

After six months post-stroke, I do pause to give thanks and celebrate successes—which is encouraged for all stroke survivors.

I've been fortunate, combining good medical care with strong personal effort to be rewarded with encouraging results. Immediately after my stroke event, Bobby got me to the emergency ward quickly and Dr Sales authorised a thrombolysis—the clot busting medication known to improve blood flow and reduce tissue damage to organs. Critically, it needs to be administered in the first four-hours post-stroke, a window I was well within. Subsequently, I also received excellent care, from doctors and nurses, and the teams of physiotherapists were inspirational, getting me to believe regaining my mobility was possible, and guiding me, with enthusiasm, careful instruction and no-nonsense compassion, to get me there.

My physical restoration continues—remembering the mantra, *recovery has no end date*. I practice strengthening exercises mixing dumbbells, therabands and treadmills with garden spades, hiking boots and swimming trunks, knowing pleasurable activities are necessary supplements to benefit body, mind and spirit, as in any formal exercise programme.

These enjoyable pastimes at slower pace, along with soothing music (an Apple iMusic subscription is a great investment), quality reading material and online courses (for discussing another time) keep my mind engaged, inspired and interested in intriguing subjects to placate any niggles and debilities from complaining muscles.

Nearly thirty years ago, Robert McCrum, English author and editor, had a debilitating stroke, at age 42. In his book, *My Year Off—Recovering Life After a Stroke*, he describes the personal impact of having a brain assault:

"It is an event that goes to the core of who and what you are, the You-ness of you. First of all, the event happens in your brain which is, without becoming unduly philosophical, the command centre of the self. Your brain is you: your moods, your skills, your character, your intelligence, your emotions, your self-expression, your self. When all that fails, you are left with the question: what was the cause? The doctors can answer questions about blood and veins and arteries and cholesterol, but that, as a friend of mine put it so aptly, is 'just the plumbing'. You —the you that's survived this upheaval within —are still left with the question: why? Before you can begin to get to why? you have to ask yourself: what? What was it that I went through? What is its significance?

What does it mean? These are questions which bring us inexorably back to Why?"

Decades on, and after a productive post-stroke career and full family life, McCrum continues to write and publish. His words still ring true, the medical profession still doesn't know when a stroke will strike or why it hits one person and not another.

Medical equipment can pinpoint the location of the impact zone, and doctors can work wonders by intervening with pre- and post-stroke surgery to unblock arteries and veins, as well as prescribe medication to keep these 'pipes' clean, but they still cannot say why a person succumbs to a stroke when they do.

Their best shot at prediction is a set of risk factors. Age and gender are two that apply to me—75% of strokes occur in people over the age of 65, especially among males—ever punctual I didn't wait long, I was 66!

Of other risk factors, like high blood pressure, dicky heart, high cholesterol, diabetes, obesity, sleep apnea and smoking, none apply to me.

I was fit, active, slim, a moderate alcohol drinker (1 standard drink a week, less after the stroke), a lifetime non-smoker, not a recreational drug user and for years I've eaten a healthy, nutritious diet with little saturated fat. My only food weakness a chunk of cheese in the evening—far from excessive. Genetically too, I have no stroke history on either side of my biological family.

When considering biology or lifestyle, I wasn't high risk pre-stroke. Yet I was struck, bang . . . out of the blue. *'Unlucky'*, my GP's assessment.

Now that I understand, through personal experience, what a stroke is and what it has done to my brain and body, I'm still, not unlike McCrum, and many other stroke survivors, drawn to why?

It's human nature to be curious. Reflecting on my life journey and how I managed key events and stress points, I can now nominate factors that possibly contributed to the *why?* I'll explore these further when returning to my memoir writing that was temporarily paused after my stroke.

As Bobby turns to sketching and drawing for her mindful practices, so I turn to writing—reflecting to understand, absorb and then step on with day-to-day life. Being able to convey life experiences into words is, once done, as soothing and revitalising as a hug, fine meal or an evening sunset.

Presently, I know three people who are undergoing treatment to combat life-threatening diseases and three more, as stroke survivors, who continue with rehab programs to restore their limb function and mobility. To them, and their close supports, I extend my good wishes. Persevere, be hopeful and embrace self-care. Believe in, and befriend, the healing qualities of the mind, body and spirit as this triad holds restorative power.

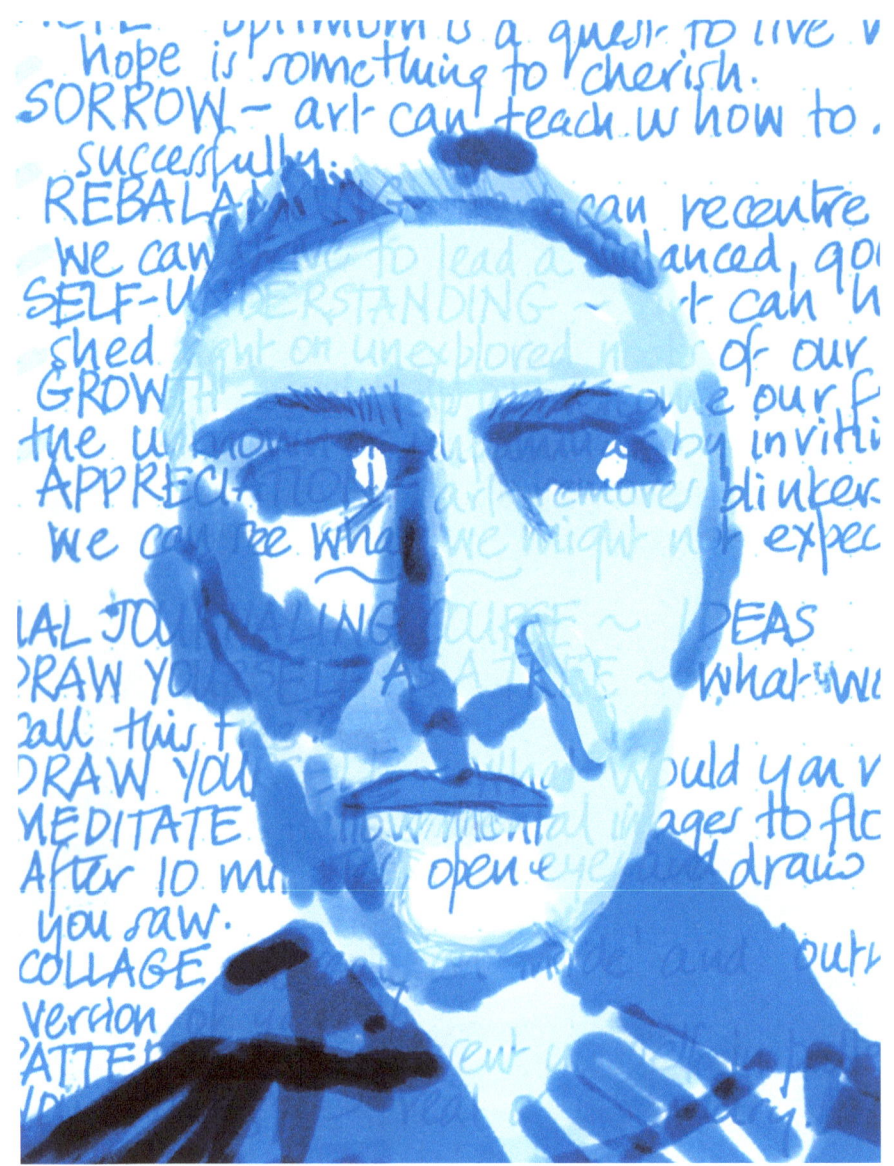

Post-Stroke Blues
Awarded First Prize
Artist Society of Canberra
Spring Exibition 2023

Part three
Ongoing recovery: body, mind and spirit

Poetry inspired by sit spotting in nature, once I'd begun the Ecotherapy Course.

DAY TWO HUNDRED AND SEVENTY-THREE

Monday, 29 January 2024
Front garden, Bonner, ACT

Sweet, Green Sit Spot

Cackling kookaburras greet the day,
soothing accompaniment to a rising sun.

Up high,
float wisps of cloud,
shifting depth perspectives to open sky.
Layers of blue, white and green unfold before my eyes,
branches alive with green summer leaves.

Stillness settles,
momentarily broken by screeches that jar,
cockatoos have their place here too.

The pink ice protea, once a sapling,
a giant two metres high, oval flower-heads aplenty,
a screen filled with sweet abundance and velvet touch.

A solitary wattlebird,
protective of its nectar-filled protea larder,
swoops on feathered intruders who dare to share the sugary patch.

Garden colours,
clustered layers of whites, blues, yellows and purple hues,
soft whites, courtesy of Gaura,

impressions of whirling butterflies,
befriended by attentive collecting bees on their daily pollen run.
Trumpet-faced blue Convolvulus,
bright yellow Gazina, greet the sunlight.
The Sweet Pea shrub alive with a purple glow,
alongside a healthy Erica, fine flowering, happily bright.

Once a bare plot,
abundant now with floral life, planted by own hands in fertile soil.
There's more . . .
an inner double row of roses, names lost in time,
a Graham Thomas among them,
full-faced, fragrant golden-yellow petals.

One and all salvaged from Bingle St,
our demolished asbestos-ridden home.
Each transplanted rose continues to flourish,
post annual August prune,
sitting beside blue pots,
gifted palettes of annual pansies, petunias,
lush Californian poppies.

I sit,
admiring my modest, colour-blessed, suburban front garden,
open to the street.

A pair of crimson Rosellas suspend their flight,
pausing briefly on their day of togetherness.

A short being-here-now practice stills the mind,
preparatory sensory awareness, welcoming a new day.
The final sip of Earl Grey tea, a notice to relinquish observation,
and leave my vibrant, sweet, green sit spot.

DAY TWO HUNDRED AND EIGHTY-EIGHT

Tuesday, 13 February 2024
Front garden, Bonner, ACT

Bare Feet

Bare feet embedded in wood bark
grounded in Mother Earth
igniting a pulse of energy
circulating through muscle and bone

Bare feet planted among roses
beneath the ash standing strong
soothing, sensual sensations
settling into inner calm

Bare feet rooted in stillness
touching skin, scanning mood
aliveness attuned to soil
breath breathing universal air

Bare feet transplanted in nature
embracing soles and toes
alert to unfolding impressions
emerging light, brings the dawn.

DAY TWO HUNDRED AND EIGHTY-NINE

Wednesday, 14 February 2024
Front garden, Bonner, ACT

Agitation

The wind has shifted,
now northerly,
strong.

Treetops swirling,
restless branches,
mimic agitation of mind.

What is it today
that brings this unsettling?
Breathe deep.

The wind blows,
stronger now,
let it shift the unsettling.

DAY TWO HUNDRED AND NINETY-TWO

Saturday, 17 February 2024
Honeysuckle Campground, Namadgi, Brindabella Ranges, ACT

Fireside Friendships

Amongst the gumtrees
fire glows
burning logs
embers grilling griddles of salmon.
Mushroom rice, salad, in waiting
sparkling water, Bentspoke & Riesling
ascent to Legoland complete.

Amongst the gumtrees
beneath a full moon
hidden by cloud
wallabies nibble bush delights
comfortable with human presence.

Amongst the gumtrees
tents erect, swags unfurled
conversation flows
the week's events in focus
fresh beginnings, a new career for Louis

in service to others.

Amongst the gumtrees
enjoyment, a communal meal
friendship shared
father, son and close mates
kindled, by warmth of flame
embraced, beneath night sky
echoing, millennia of fireside friendships.

(Thanks to Louis, Sandy & Danny)

DAY TWO HUNDRED AND NINETY-FOUR

Monday, 19 February 2024
Aslings Beach, Eden, NSW

Wagga On My Mind

Bare feet
soft granular sand underfoot.

Log sitting
watching the incoming tide.

Good to be back
how long has it been?

Eighteen months, perhaps more
since the sight and scent of sea.

The soothing sounds of ocean
seagulls aplenty, feeding in mid-air.

Between the ebb and flow of tumbling waves
Wagga comes to mind.

*Twenty-five years since arriving
to a new country, offering a fresh start.*

*Familiar southern seasons
summer lingering into February.*

*The Southern Cross, known constellation
a real marker of belonging.*

*What stories do I have of continuity
of living, to bring me home to self?*

DAY TWO HUNDRED AND NINETY-FIVE

Tuesday, 20 February 2024
Forest Bathing, Cotter River Bend, ACT

Befriending an Oak

Four ancient cork oaks
stand tall
soak in sunlight.
A century plus of filtering
to release fresh air
for my
our
daily benefit.

Their chunky skins of cushioned bark
a shield against bushfires
like the myelin sheaths
protecting the nerve endings
within my body
under repair.

The pons
at the base of my skull
starved of oxygen

when struck by stroke
suspended mobility to right-sided limbs.

Laid low
the daily challenge
exercise
to get back on my feet
to walk.

To regain arm, hand, finger movement
to feed, clean, dress, drive,
to touch.

I sit
drawn to rest the back of my head
against the noble oak
soaking its energy
to restore inner strength.

To stand tall
patient
trusting
vital once more, with life
as is my woody friend.

DAY TWO HUNDRED AND NINETY-SIX

Wednesday, 21 February 2024

Ecotherapy Course, second online group meeting

Anticipation

We gather virtually
via Zoom
from across the country
overseas too.

Communal desire for connection
to reconnect with nature.
Find our ecological selves
green our consciousness.

To come home to self
swap ego with eco sensibility.
Open to discovery, natural growth
to share with each other.

What comes alive when attentive to nature?
When observing with quiet intent?
Watching our world unfold
where do our minds, our bodies and spirit sit?

*Awakening our senses
to learn a new multi-sensory
multi-species language.
Integrate the messaging
decipher non-verbal cues.*

*Less thinking mind
more intentional awareness
enhances connection.*

*Attuned to visual metaphors,
memory lines
nature igniting deeper consciousness.
Channelled through body, heart and spirit
open to seeing
listening
feeling
somatic sensation.*

*Remembering our mentors
Roszak, Macy, Jordan & Young.*

*At times it's hard to find the stillness
to settle into a spotting mindset.
Keeping the body alert, comfortable, agreeable to be still,
curbing the itch to stretch or move.*

*Thoughts emerge, distractions
Am I worthy, good enough?
How to process the chaos in me?
Is it safe to be vulnerable?*

Passivity, what to do with that?
Self-sabotage, will it raise its head again?
This road, is it worth travelling?
Where is the learning?
Perhaps, impatience kicks in.

In opening up
the senses find their spot.
In seeing, we notice
clouds, birds, rustling leaves
hear cicadas sing,
touch raindrops
feel the shifting wind.

Perspective alters
expansiveness grows
perception sharpens.

Time pauses . . .
Now becomes.
It's all that matters.
Momentarily, we sit in awe
and wonder
observing . . .

Doing it our way
the woodpecker, finches and cicadas speak
we hug our pets, nurture pot plants, garden
wander through forests, sand dunes
admire the ocean
sensing
embracing the abundance of eco-wisdom.

(With thanks to: Amanda, Amelia, Cassie, Charlotte, David, Geoff, Hayden, Laura, Leah, Louise, Maddie, Mirjam, Rachael, Rhiannon, Sarah & Seth.)

DAY THREE HUNDRED AND FOUR

Thursday, 29 February 2024
Front garden, Bonner, ACT

Leap Year

Bright sunny morning
blue sky,
brushes of white cloud
bees collecting pollen.

Vapour jet trails, flight lines,
the first planes of day.
Cockatoos gliding overhead, screeching,
ash leaves hint of changing colour.

Neighbours driving off to work
earth drilling in building development nearby.
A magpie's song
melodious rhythms announcing a new day.

Another day
the moon, earth and sun spinning in orbit.
The bees, birds and branches in natural flow
oblivious to the extra calendar day.

*Nature, unfolds naturally, regardless of calendars,
constructs in celestial time control.
Almanacs dissolve, lose their rigidity,
open to continuity, existence, I embrace another day.*

DAY THREE HUNDRED AND EIGHTEEN

Thursday, 14 March 2024
Adelaide Botanic Gardens

Changing Seasons

Singular leaves
Detach
float
gravity's pull
thirty-five metres to the ground.

Each leaf's moment of release
nature's rhythmic
spontaneous course
after a summer of soaking sun
cleansing air
providing shade,
shelter.

At what moment in autumn's first light
do individual leaves decide to fall
to drift down to earth
settle on the ground
among kindred leaves?

Life
full summer bloom
before each fall
then rest
to await another spring.

DAY THREE HUNDRED AND TWENTY-SEVEN

Saturday, 23 March 2024
Forest Bathing, Tidbinbilla Nature Reserve, ACT

Double Delight

Drawn
to a single tree
to sit
within the eucalyptus forest.

Place of quiet
giving attention
seeing
feeling
what arises,
without
and within.

In sight
a single trunk
mighty Peppermint
forty metres skywards
halo of sunlight
embracing the green,
overarching canopy.

*Decades of seasoned growth
ancestral witness
to storms
fire
blissful calm days
branches holding memories
cradling shedded sheaths
of discarded bark.*

*Time lapses
passing thoughts
come
go.*

*Shifting shadows
lightness of breeze
distant flow
a running creek
bird calls.
I stand
walk to one side
cast eyes upwards
Surprise . . .
this giant peppermint
has twin towering trunks,
not one!*

*Shifting position
changes perspective,
a new reality
emerges
from different sight lines.*

Expansion of vision
one becomes two
more to see
observe
double the delight :)

(National Eucalyptus Day with thanks for Julie & Holly)

DAY THREE HUNDRED AND TWENTY-SEVEN

Saturday, 23 March 2024
Full moon, Kurrajong Point, Weston Park, ACT

Lunar Readings

On the lake's edge, beneath mature pines
We gather in welcoming spirit

To collect water, offer blessing
Infuse liquid life force with love and respect

With intention, song, poetry and praise
To purify, cleanse, undo what's been done

Healing vibrations, to clean, bring clarity
Returning our watery life force, to source, to flow

Along its lengthy path into the Murrumbidgee
Onwards to the Murray and Southern Ocean

Joined momentarily by River Man
Thanking us, dissolving back into spiritual form

Sparkling waters, golden sunset, ending day
Night enters, emblazoned by brightness of rising moon

Thoughts and words spoken for a wounded friend
Collective love, support, willed her way

A meal—soup, bread, pie, carrots, guacamole, tea
Shared in communion, joyous conversation

Partnered by full-faced, bold and beautiful moon
Delivering rays of ancient wisdom, ancestral belonging

Spirit embodying our wholeness, peace within
To appreciate, commit to protecting our vulnerable world.

(With thanks to the Moon, Julie, Kay, Liz & Lynne)

DAY THREE HUNDRED AND THIRTY-FOUR

Saturday, 30 March 2024
Front garden, Bonner, ACT

Misty Dawn

First mist
mysterious light
Trees, bushes, plants
in silhouette
Diluted visual form

A single, silken thread
spider unseen
Crossing gutter above
to Rose, to Rose
Tip of Guara stem, to Rose
across to Erica bush green

A single, silken thread
loosely spanned
Firmly fixed
to points of intersection
Temporary connections
pathway to somewhere

I breathe outwards, towards the thread
it remains still
Closer, a second breath
the thread unmoved in suspension
My breath weaves over, around
dissolves into thin air

A gentle breeze rises
the thread sways along its path
Moved by nature
unmoved by human breath
Small mystery

First misty morning
feet embedded in wood bark
Acute visual observation
interrupted by arriving Rosellas
Replacing feeding bees
winged to sweeter nectar

A day passes
dawn, sunlight emerges
Mist and silky thread gone
Ephemeral connections
served their purpose
The spider
still unseen.

DAY THREE HUNDRED AND FORTY-EIGHT
Saturday, 13 April 2024
Garden Chair, Bonner, ACT

First Mist

Mysterious mist, adorns the air
amidst early morning light
Autumn's first
thicker, forming fog
lower down the street.

Stocking feet embedded in wood bark
Woollen top, hat, added warmth
thermals against the temperature drop

The mist softens hard lines
of houses, streetlamps
the leafless winter trees
standing in silhouette
past greenery figments of imagination

Seasonal change drifts in
the last rose blooms
farewell summer's vibrant palette

Replaced by proteas
Pink blooms aplenty
Absorbing fresh sunlight

How tall the protea bush?
So healthy, two metres plus
Must love its sun-filled spot
as I do, sit spotting
welcoming the dawn
in the company of birdsong

The chorus, in emerging light,
opens nature's rhythm to a new day
Momentarily, stillness within
sits beside me, inner nature
blending with true nature
a touch of blissfulness.

FIRST ANNIVERSARY OF STROKE

Thursday, 2 May 2024
Sit Spot Garden Chair, Bonner, ACT

Becoming One

Morning sunlight shines upon me
Rays penetrate the leafless ash tree.
Absorbing the warmth
I'm nourished by life-giving light.

One year, post-stroke
I'm alive, mobile.
Capable of independent living,
steady, sturdy, embracing life.

I count my blessings
speech, cognition, memory, intuition intact.
Slower right-sided limb movement
a reminder pace of life is important,
for balance, harmony, longer life.

Thanks to the medical team, family, friends, pets,
to Nature, for being there when needed.
To Self for opening awareness, to greater consciousness

of the importance of life,
of being, less of repetitive doing.

Busyness, devoid of care for others,
for Self excessive doing exposes vulnerabilities to hostile attack,
health fails, wellbeing suffers, wholeness is lost.

Enter recovery, encompassing the physical, psychological,
spiritual and relational domains of daily living.
Returning to vitality, consciousness, to being fully alive,
I rise and walk on, with Nature and patience by my side.

Stroke—the strike bringing me to my senses.

DAY THREE HUNDRED AND SIXTY-NINE

Monday, 6 May 2024
Garden chair, Bonner, ACT

Statin Intolerance

Brown leaves roll across the ground
Propelled by gusty winds

Back and forth
A turbulent tide of fallen growth

Another wave skips forward
And back, in restless agitation

Mirroring thoughts of mine
Bodily intolerance to statins

Intolerable muscle ache
Seeping, sweeping through my limbs

The bare tree limbs sway in rhythm
Sensing my unease, inner disturbance

My churning within, finds an ally
The fallen leaves roll on, back and forth

A decision needs to be made
how much longer do I endure this discomfort

There must be an alternative way to wellness
Tomorrow, I stop the medication

Continue meditation, healthy eating, exercise
Restful sleep, sit spotting, self compassion

To embed calmness, balance, equanimity
To body, for mind, within spirit, supporting my well-being.

(After a doctor's appointment, a week before, where he recommended I return to statin medication. I did for a week, but the adverse side effects returned, my whole body filled with muscle pain and discomfort. Since then, I no longer take the medication).

DAY THREE HUNDRED AND EIGHTY-FIVE

Tuesday, 21 May 2024
Front Garden, Bonner, ACT

First Frost

Icicles
glow white on
woodchip, parked cars, roof tiles
crispy chill
amid sparkling morning light.

The sun's arc shifted
lowering to north
Its rays breaking through
bare ash branches
Seed pods hanging on
tiny lanterns, seed dispersed.

-2 degrees
stocking feet embedded in wood bark
body warmed, under woolies
blanketed legs, head beneath bush hat
My breath illuminated
bursts of vapour, dissolving into air.

Rhythm of life
cup of Lady Grey
welcome warmth, savouring hot brew
Attention given to nature
any communal friends?

The resident wattlebird
probes his beak
between bracts, seeking pollen anthers
within the blooming proteas
His morning brew
gathered from 'Pink Ice' flowers

The blanket of ice crystals
marks seasonal change
Winter arriving
the morning chill
on ears, nose and fingers, enlivening
The sensory touch
good to feel, head to toe
Body, spirit fully alive.

DAY THREE HUNDRED AND EIGHTY-SEVEN

Thursday, 23 May 2024
Garden chair, Night Sky, Bonner, ACT

Anniversary Moon

Moonbeams fill the night sky
courtesy of full moon
gleaming bright

A circular mirror of pure,
white light
wholesome reflected sunlight

The bright disc
gradually rises
behind the neighbour's house

The bare ash tree
cast in silhouette
a canopy of connecting threads

A giant cosmic x-ray
of arteries, veins, capillaries
In filtered outline

Feeds the pulse of being
heartened by the glow
I count blessings

For life, mobility, good health
Tonight
in the chillness of autumn night

We celebrate our 26th wedding anniversary
warmed by familiar vintage
Cape Pinotage

The gift of partnership
companionship runs deep
cyclical patterns of togetherness

The glow of moonbeams
momentarily bring
certainty to an uncertain world.

(Bobby in Broken Hill enjoying an Art Retreat)

DAY THREE HUNDRED AND NINETY-SIX

Saturday, 15 June 2024
Front garden, Bonner, ACT

Nature's Maxim

Be Patient
Trust
Enjoy

DAY THREE HUNDRED AND NINETY-SEVEN

Monday, 16 June 2024
Among the trees, Canberra Centenary Track

Hall to Home

Back on the Centenary Track
Hall village to Bonner home
16km walk, last done
fourteen months ago.

Crispy, frosty, winter morning
Clear sunny day
Ideal for having a go
test strength, endurance
for right leg in post-stroke recovery.

The path glistens
puddles from rain past
In shadow patches, lie morning dew
Icy to touch.

Upwards, to One Tree Hill
beacon marking a future Capital
Circular basin, lined with hills

the Brindabella ranges
Water catchment for the city.

Six kms in, I sit among the Yellow Box
On a hilly knoll, boundary fence alongside
Alone among green friends
Reflecting on life since
sitting here last, more than a year ago.

Stroke, hospital, rehabilitation of right-sided limbs
farewelling old Thomas, rebuilding the new
over weeks, months, a year plus.
I delight in restored mobility
walking freely in nature, under sunlight
blue skies, in forests and grasslands green.

Moving on, along
up, down
hills, slopes.
Close encounters with wallabies
family mobs lie close among the trees.
Hazel eyes glow bright
greeting, recognition
I leave them to their slumber.

Ten kms in I stop, off track
my favourite tree.
Two hundred plus years living.
Solid, earthed, standing strong
An inspiration to me.

*Back home
milestone complete
tender hip and muscles
in need of night's rest.*

*My footsteps left on track
meeting those of yesteryear.
This interlude of illness
a memory left in the past
The present strives for wellness.*

DAY FOUR HUNDRED AND TWO

Friday, 21 June 2024
Himalayan Cedar Forest, Arboretum, ACT

Winter Solstice

We assemble in the carpark
alongside the Himalayan Cedar forest
its century living roots embedded
in the landscape, flourishing.

Volunteers, we've come to wrap
tree trunks with knitted woollen scarves
the annual Warm Trees ritual
coinciding with the winter solstice.

With bags of knitted scarfs and cable ties
we disperse into the evergreen grove
wrapping 'timber of the gods'
so young.

Their life expectancy
another half a millennium long
given we protect
look after, our natural environment.

Time drifts, stills
the traffic drones along Tugger's Parkway
audibly softened, as attention shifts to
enfolding rings of woollen warmth.

Nature swaddling
round and round limbs of furrowed bark
tuning ourselves, sharing our warmth
to honour natural flow of existence.

Point of transition
to pause
anticipate what is to come
days progressing towards more sunlight.

A turning, resting in the interlude
of cold with darkness
knowing light with warmth
is on its way.

ONE YEAR, TWO MONTHS

Tuesday, 2 July 2024
Home, Bonner, ACT

Pathways to Physical Restoration: Body, Mind, Heart and Spirit

Pausing to reflect on my post-stroke journey, the message is clear: my physical recovery continues; it's ongoing, a steady progression, requiring patience and daily practice.

The assault on my brain was a major blow that, over the past 14 months, has challenged my physical, mental, emotional and spiritual capabilities.

Any illness or injury I experienced in the past—and thankfully there haven't been many—healed within weeks. None, like this stroke, required an ongoing whole-of-being emphasis to regain what was lost. In my current circumstances, to restore my physical movement, build strength, stamina and endurance, while keeping my sanity and shape future aspirations.

I'm lucky, fortunate, blessed. I've managed to restore my primary limb function and many of my finer motor skills through intensive exercise—a combination of physiotherapy and engaging in multiple activities of daily living. Although the muscles remain weak, I'm capable of independent living. The ability of the brain to rewire itself, prompted by physical stimuli of repetitive movement, is a wonder of biology and human life.

Prior to my stroke, I enjoyed complete able-bodiedness. It was part of my identity. I had no bodily barriers to active living. I completed household chores, diverse work tasks, played sport and engaged in recreational pastimes with physical ease.

Having to relearn how to perform basic movement, to teach my right-sided limbs to function normally again, has been a challenge. One I accepted without complaint, driven by a primal desire to get my mobility back, as my quality of life depended on it.

I remember sitting in a wheelchair in rehab hospital exercising my right arm, wrist and hand to revive their function. My arm rested on a table, I tried to move it in a ninety-degree arc and back again. It felt like a dead weight. The first attempts at the repetitive movement took enormous willpower and energy. As did my wrist, when placed over a rolled towel, my forearm resting on a table, to affect the simple action of lifting it up and down, for five and up to ten repetitions. Straightforward, but so hard.

Slightly easier, though stranger to experience, was the tingling of an electric shock in my hand and fingers, delivered by a FES device wired to my forearm, to induce nerve and muscle impulses. The charge, when switched on and off, prompted my hand to involuntarily open and close.

Day after day I practiced simple exercises, multiple times, to instruct my brain to set up new neural connections to ignite and improve basic limb movement:

- picking up small wooden pins with my fingertips and placing them into the holes of a peg board. Removing the pegs from the board and starting again, and again;
- using tweezers to pick up small plastic beads to drop them into a saucer alongside. Repeat, again and again.
- learning to pick up marbles and balance the balls on top of golf tees stuck into a container lid. Repeat, again and again;

- when my wrist and finger control returned, to hold a pen and practice handwriting, slowly and shakily writing the alphabet in a notebook, over and over again. The highlight, writing my full name, for the first time, post-stroke;
- practicing my touch-typing skills, one and two fingers at first, slowly progressing to nimble fingered typing with both hands. Such an important skill for opening communication to family, friends and the broader world, via the internet; and
- holding a knife to cut a role of play putty to build my wrist and hand strength, allowing me to progress to a vegetable peeler, to skin a potato, and to feed myself at the dinner table, holding a knife and fork, like Bobby does.

Simple functional movements we take for granted, yet necessary for engaging in the activities of daily living—for standard functioning, for maintaining our dignity.

Similarly, I've had to practice standing up, walking and other exercises, to strengthen my weakened right leg, stiffened ankle, foot and toes. To find my feet, hold my balance, improve my gait and stride, bring flexibility back into my ankle, freely lift my toes and incrementally, extend my walking distance.

I regularly alternate my exercise routines between upper and lower limbs and for whole-of-body balance, and work my left side to keep its functional conditioning.

Repetitive and focused exercise is important for regaining movement, so that it becomes more precise, quicker, stronger and ideally, mimics natural ease. Whenever an exercise becomes too easy, a change is made, to make it more difficult, or to bring in a new one, for variety, to continue to improve functional control and build strength. Variety is important, and I've been fortunate to mix and match between weights, walking, swimming, stretching, gardening and domestic chores.

Into my second post-stroke year, ongoing exercise is still an important practice for physical recovery. Formal physiotherapy sessions are essential, yet alone are insufficient to regain and sustain, full functional mobility. Additional and regular, whole-of-body physical movement is needed for mastering finer control.

Household chores, vacuuming the carpet, dusting furniture, washing the windows, hanging up the washing and preparing meals have played their part in me regaining and strengthening my finer motor skills. Importantly, also to build confidence, and bring purpose, to reengage with basic routines of home life. Some of these tasks, for example, hanging clothes on the outside wash line or dusting the cornices inside the house, help build my flexibility, greater reach and strength in shoulder and arm movements, as they stimulate neurons for function required above head height.

Today, the attributes of my physical abilities that bring me joy and satisfaction, are my abilities to brush my teeth, shave with a wet razor, rub shampoo into my scalp, button my shirt, tie my shoe laces, use a knife and fork, peel vegetables, carry a cup of tea in each hand without spilling either, peg clothes onto the top of the wash line, sweep with broom in hand, change my bed linen, wash the ute, prune roses, touch type and use a power drill. Basic personal and household tasks, once temporarily lost, their return a boost to my agency and an enabler for independence.

With my love of the outdoors, more inviting exercise is being able to walk in nature and the garden again. In my first few days in hospital, when 'walking' implied being suspended in a harness above a treadmill or shuffling 10, 20 or 50 steps with a minder either side. The desire to feast my eyes on the green Brindabella Mountains, through the window at the end of the corridor, infused each step with purpose. The sight of those southern mountains gave me an inspirational charge for restoring my mobility so that I could get back into nature, long my spiritual home.

This feeling for nature, I recall, was further aroused when wheeled on a stretcher, out into the Canberra winter air, and into an ambulance to transport me to the rehab hospital nearby. That icy chill of sub-zero air was absolute bliss. It affirmed that nature—as comforting life force—remained present and accessible, despite being hit by stroke.

Settling into the rehab hospital for intensive physiotherapy, I was one of few who insisted wheeling myself into the courtyard gardens to get my daily dose of sunlight and fresh air in the presence of plants.

A couple of months after returning home, I set out to finish a garden project I'd begun pre-stroke. I'd built two wooden veggie containers on our sidewalk, to make use of the northerly aspect that provided full sun. Over a couple of days, with the help of Sandy and Louis, we hitched the box trailer to my ute to drive to Corkhill's to collect loads of forest litter and soil. Over many days thereafter, I manually shovelled the rich veggie mix into the 1.5 x 1.5 x 0.9-centimetre containers in 15-, 30- or 60-minute sessions.

Bobby and I also purchased three half wine-barrels, made from high quality oak, that were delivered to our door. I sanded and varnished each one, before filling them with soil and planting a variety of herbs in two, and a small lemon tree in one. A couple of weeks later, when walking outside to water the garden, I noticed roving cockatoos had decimated the herb garden and decapitated the stem of the blossoming lemon tree!

We repurchased and replanted replacements and I set about building covers, from black nylon netting, left over from my cat enclosure building days as Mr Petman, to provide protective covers for each of the plant containers.

These tasks, which would have taken me three days to complete pre-stroke, took me three months to finish post-stroke. A sign of how much slower and weaker I'd become following my brain assault. The positives, the project contributed to building my strength and confidence. Importantly, it gave me pleasure and since then we have enjoyed a summer crop of home-grown vegetables. The winter planting is also doing well.

My mental fortitude was tested during the first six months of recovery when having to deal with bouts of extreme weariness. The unfamiliar sensation usually occurred after a walk or working in the garden. The feeling sent alarm bells swirling through my mind—was it the onset of another stroke, or just a passing phase of brain fatigue?

These unsettling moments prompted an immediate reaction—I'd say the alphabet aloud to myself to hear if my speech was slurred. And following that, stretch both my arms at ninety degrees, and hold them there for a few seconds, noticing whether they were inclined to droop, showing signs of weakness. Often, I'd repeat these manual tests, and once satisfied there was no change in bodily function, I'd sit quietly, compose myself, and focus on my breathing.

The thought of having another stroke was unnerving—statistically the possibility is 1 in 4. Over time, I've realised the strange felt sensation was simply tiredness. My brain fatigued after having to work intensely to maintain the demand for functional body movements. Fortunately, these bouts of fatigue have occurred less and less as my stamina and strength have improved.

Walking has long been a passion, especially in beautiful natural surroundings. Living in Canberra, we're blessed with abundant natural landscape. In our suburb of Bonner, along its northern edge, lie natural corridors of wooded bushland that offer many pathways for walking. I regularly take walks into this bushland, a favourite the 3km return stroll to Golden Sun Moth lookout. Occasionally, progressing further up the hill, onto the most northern section of the Canberra Centenary Trail—the latter a 145km track encircling the city—for a southerly view over our garden city.

Once the doctor cleared me to drive—three months after my stroke—my world expanded with the freedom to venture out to other favourite local walking tracks, around Yerrabi Pond, in Mulligan's Flats and the Cork Forest at the National Arboretum. These walks improved my walking performance, extending distance and increasing speed, the latter less important to me than the distance covered.

Gradually, over the months, I increased my walking range from 100m, 200m, 500m to a kilometre and more. I'm now comfortable with regular 2km to 4km walks and have managed the iconic 5km Bridge to Bridge in the Parliamentary Triangle and, a month ago, Hall to home, a 16km walk, along the Centenary Track, which I'd last done 14 months previously. A personal post-stroke best, for mind and body. In addition to extending my range, these walks bring me the satisfaction of edging closer to my pre-stroke physical ability. I have a way to go, especially if I want to carry a backpack for multiple day and overnight hikes—achieving these goals is probably many months away.

Returning to the Gungahlin Leisure Centre to swim in the indoor 50m pool was another activity I looked forward to. Swimming, once or twice a week, brings novelty to my exercise programme, as it works my body differently, and being in water both clears my mind and refreshes my spirit.

Nine weeks after my stroke, Bobby and I went to the pool for the first time. When entering the water, via the poolside steps, the sensory rush to my body was startling—I tingled from head to toe. I'd lost my ability to swim, my coordination completely haphazard. All I could do was jump on the spot and splash my arms to the side.

Over successive weekly pool visits, I slowly transformed from drunk frog to novice swimmer, as my brain relearnt the signalling for creating the physical movements required for backstroke, breaststroke and crawl. In recent months, my swimming ability has returned, although not as fluid as pre-stroke due to my weakened right leg.

I've written before that stroke recovery is as much mental as it is physical. It requires constant commitment and effort, drawing down on mental as well as physical capacity. This fact was highlighted early on when, during my second week in rehab hospital, I attended an online information session in the dining room. Simone Dorsch, Associate Professor in Physiotherapy at the Australian Catholic University, interviewed two stroke survivors, Brian Beh and Stephanie Ho.

Brian had survived a severe stroke seven years previously, at age 68, and Steph, 13 years before, at the age of 22. They spoke openly and encouragingly about their own post-stroke recovery having started with extreme physical impairment, which in the case of Steph, also involved speech loss. Both had restored their full mobility, through sustained physiotherapy, to return to able-bodied functional living.

Listening to their personal stories of perseverance was inspiring and empowering. Akin to Elyse, my first physiotherapist's invitation, "Let's go for a walk, Tom" when she met me on my second day in Calvary Hospital. Her words instilled a sense of self-belief that my damaged body was repairable. I could restore function by taking that first step.

Brian and Steph highlighted that there was no endpoint to recovery. As stroke survivors, we need to remain active and exercise daily. The aim is to get our muscles working with sufficient intensity, and frequency of movement, to challenge our bodies and minds to strive for functional improvement, no matter how small. This process requires a mental shift, to find determination and motivation, for sustaining long term physical exercise.

I tapped into my memory of having twice run an ultramarathon—the 56km Two Oceans Ultramarathon, in 1988 and 1992, in Cape Town. In addition, I'd run other standard marathons and completed long distance hikes, over multiple days, carrying a 20kg backpack, the most recent four years ago, along the Tarkine Coast in Tasmania in 2020.

Knowing I'd trained for physical endurance events in the past, and my most recent work activity—building 400+ cat enclosures in suburban backyards, over six years—secured an inner confidence that I had the mental capacity to endure a long, physical challenge. Being older in age, a minor hindrance, not a handicap.

The one unknown, would my post-stroke weakened body sustain intensive sessions of physiotherapy over a long period? It hasn't faltered—not once has it failed to respond or keep up with the physical exercise—and for that I'm most grateful.

To sharpen my mental resilience, I did what I've often done, and that is to search for quality courses online to improve my knowledge base. Feeding my mind with quality and reliable information about health and wellbeing, I believed would help me better plan, pace and perform my recovery journey.

Importantly, I wanted to keep personal agency for what lay ahead, so I could take responsibility for reversing my impaired mobility—a goal I aspired to and am eager to work towards.

At the end of June 2023, I looked at The Great Courses—a teaching company providing educational resources via packaged lectures, available online, presented by specialists in their field. Having sourced their courses in the past, notably during COVID lockdowns, I knew their value as quality learning tools which I could complete in my own time at home. Two packages appealed to me, *Building Your Resilience: Finding Meaning in Adversity*, comprising 24 half-hour lectures, presented by Molly Birkholm, an internationally renowned trauma specialist, yoga and mindfulness teacher. And the second, *Mind-Body Medicine: The New Science of Optimal Health*, a programme of 36 half-hour lectures, written and delivered by Professor Jason Satterfield from the University of California, San Francisco.

Over the next couple of months, I watched the full suite of lectures, across both courses, finding the content engaging and enjoyable, akin to mental exercise for my intellect, to complement the daily physical exercise I required of my body. I was drawn to Satterfield's holistic health philosophy—long a view of mine—that to manage our health in general and repair our bodies after a medical emergency in particular, we need to look at the whole person and how we interact with our environment in developing strategies and practices to restore and sustain better health. His succinct framing of the biopsychosocial model of health care—*'what makes us sick, what makes us well, and what we can do about it'*—resonated deeply with me.

I was equally impressed by Molly Birkholm's knowledge, personal experience and delivery style, so much so, I purchased a second course of hers, *iRest: Integrative Restoration Yoga Nidra for Deep Relaxation*. Based on ancient Buddhist philosophy and practice, the content focused on using guided meditation to develop skills for achieving mindful awareness and inner stillness, to enhance healthy living and wellbeing. Over many days, I watched her 24 half-hour lectures, repeating some of the most engaging.

I was interested in what both tutors said about chronic stress to better understand what effect excessive or prolonged stress had on my body, and to equip me with adapting practices to manage the adverse impacts of stressful events on my physical, mental and emotional states of being.

I highlight stress, as I've come to realise my body didn't fail me when yielding to a stroke. I let my body down by allowing myself, over decades, to become a casualty of inadequate self-care when it came to managing traumatic life events. An unhealthy pattern of bottling unsettled emotions didn't serve me well over the long term.

I was born and blessed with a fully functioning healthy body. A strong healthy body was something I had always depended on—it served me well for over six decades. My inability, however, to adequately deal with traumatic events and stressful circumstances—favouring rigid thinking and suppression of emotion as defences—meant that over decades, progressive stress built up within my body and somatically trapped within it. Without an adaptive safety valve, the accumulating stress eventually wore my system down, prompting its own release—a brain snap causing an ischemic stroke.

Prior to my brain assault, I had few red markers of a pending stroke victim, apart from my age and poor stress management.

I was fit, had a healthy heart, no high blood pressure and my cholesterol levels were within the normal range. I wasn't overweight, didn't suffer from diabetes or any other chronic disease. I followed a Mediterranean diet, slept well, had no substance dependencies— took no medication or recreational drugs and seldom had more than four standard alcoholic drinks a month. I exercised regularly, never smoked, wasn't socially isolated and had no genetic history of stroke events on either side of my biological family. I rarely suffered from illness, neither flu, the common cold, nor COVID.

Given my health card and lifestyle, of the two remaining risk factors as probable causes of my stroke, my inability to manage stress was the main factor. Prior to my brain assault, my body was constantly tense. Seldom was I physically relaxed. My jaw was perennially taut, my shoulders hunched, scalp tight, my torso rigid. I'd go to bed each night with clenched jaw and fists and wake up the same way in the morning. I had developed a permanent headache, often putting a heat pack on my neck at night to try and relieve the tension. I rushed eating meals, was perennially impatient, ever-vigilant and at times had a short fuse, especially when receiving sub-standard service. Regular exercise reduced my agitation and muscular tension, but only briefly. Long term relaxation was foreign to me.

The main suspect for creating this heightened bodily tension, was my mind, an unsettled headspace, as I habitually cogitated over life events—being adopted, superannuation finances and unscrupulous advisers, what to do in retirement, marital squabbles, the constant damage to our planet and the recent death of my mother (the latter occurring two months before my stroke).

I worried about many things silently, incessantly, with occasional verbal outbursts.

Often consumed by negative thoughts, this thinking tended to increase feelings of irritability, annoyance and disapproval. These emotions would manifest into anger, which I turned inwards, onto myself, leaving a sense of impotence even though, outwardly, I appeared happy, in control, responsive and efficient to meeting the demands and duties of daily life.

Being in such a prolonged and perpetual state of constriction—my mind agitated, my body tense, emotions unsettled—it's not surprising my healthy, strong, reliable body in response, silently decreed 'enough-is-enough'. Dramatically, it enforced its own medical emergency to reappraise my thinking, behaviours and life purpose.

In the immediate aftermath of my stroke, I noticed my jaw relaxed, and a complete absence of tension in my cheeks, scalp, throat and neck. Post-stroke my body is at ease, relaxed without tension, for the first time in years.

Meditating has helped to calm my mind, and by extension, relax my body. For the past nine months, I've been meditating regularly, almost daily. I repeat many of Birkholm's guided meditations; they've become standard practice to evoke the relaxation response, to activate my parasympathetic nervous system to reduce my breathing and heart rate, calm my mind and bring stillness within. Meditation has become a vital practice supporting my recovery, essential as physical exercise.

Through Birkholm and Satterfield, I was introduced to post-traumatic growth, a branch of positive psychology, developed in the mid 1990s, by Richard Tedeschi and Lawrence Calhoun, both Professors of Psychology at the University of North Carolina at Charlotte, USA. Their research and practicing model, a contemporary focus on the millennia old conundrum: how to understand, modulate and ease the effects of suffering? All of us, at some point in our lives, are likely to face challenges that inflict suffering on ourselves, our families or the natural world, instigated by natural disasters, serious illness, death of someone close, loss of employment, financial insecurity, even war.

In post-traumatic growth, I found a framework to guide me through adapting positively to my changed health. With my identity shaken, my physical movement impaired and emotions raw, I had to reappraise my life strategies. Clearly, what I had being doing, wasn't providing what I wanted or needed—a stroke wasn't part of my retirement plan.

The post-traumatic growth model requires personal exploration in developing new thinking and practices across five domains when struggling with highly challenging life events. The first of these is identifying, valuing and utilizing *personal strengths*. From day one, from within my inner depths, rose a determination to regain my mobility for independent living. I accepted my situation and got to work, to get better in body and mind, supported by my heart and spirit. I've been surprised and encouraged by my inner strength.

I began to investigate and experiment with new ways to better manage stressful events when I became aware that *exploring new possibilities*, was another domain of post-traumatic growth. In psychological terms, allowing myself greater mental and emotional flexibility, to change my thought patterns and express my feelings. Also, to adopt practices to support my wellbeing rather than feed tension and suppress healthy emotional ignition.

I've grasped that knowing endless theories about good health—and I've accumulated many of the years—are no substitute for the actual practice of self-care. For me, this means regular practice to reduce patterns of critical, distrustful and perfectionist thinking and in parallel, swap the suppression of uncomfortable emotions with either assertive expression, or stillness, at the appropriate time and place. Regular meditation, sit spotting, walking in nature, writing poetry and drafting this book are tangible expressions of *exploring new possibilities* to improve nurturing relationships with myself and others.

My post-stroke experience is teaching me to *improve relationships*, the third factor in post-traumatic growth. Being introverted and not wishing to draw attention to myself—a tendency compounded by the legacy of carrying a fractured identity as an adopted person— I've long known I reenergise myself by spending time outdoors in nature and engaging in solo creative pursuits. In contrast, what drains my energy reserves are frequent social engagements, surrounded by lots of people.

Beyond immediate family and close friends, my preference for privacy before people, extends to low use of social media. I have an ambivalent relationship with social media, preferring irregular face-to-face-real-life contacts than frequent telephone conversations or daily postings to online networks. I'm comfortable with using email or Messenger as communication channels for personal chats, servicing arrangements and for emergencies.

Inspired by the kindness Bobby and I received in the early phases of my recovery, when housebound, I reached out to others—to rekindle past friendships, create new ones and to reinvigorate my social interactions.

One of the first was to friend and fellow adoptee Jo-Ann Sparrow, who I'd last connected with ten years before, and only met in person six weeks before my stroke—at the 10th anniversary events held in Canberra to remember the National Apology for Forced Adoptions. For a decade, I'd been an active player in post-adoption activism and forums, including attending the national apology in Parliament House on 21 March 2013.

I'd decided to suspend my involvement in adoption matters once I ventured into a new role as Mr Petman. Nonetheless, my interest, and lifelong effects of being an adopted person remain. And in the aftermath of recovering from my stroke, and the death of my biological mother, I was drawn to speak, to share that aspect of my past, through a lengthy interview with Jo-Ann, on her *Adopt Perspective* podcast that she produces for Jigsaw Queensland. A nonprofit, post-adoption support organisation, assisting people search and reconnect with biological kin and help manage the emotional journey that follows.

Three-and-half-months post-stroke, when I sat down for the online interview, I was in an emotionally shaky and vulnerable state, dealing with the effects of my brain injury and compromised by physical impairment to my right-sided limbs. At the time, my brain was affecting my emotional regulation, as I sometimes switched from tears to laughter without control, not ideal for public performance. The interview, later posted to air, was an important stepping stone in facing my own emotional fragility, not least the feeling of having suffered another loss which adoptees are all familiar with, though find hard to articulate, let alone live with. Allowing myself the opportunity to speak, and to be heard by a sympathetic ear, smoothed a pathway for getting out and engaging in more social activities.

After I'd completed the lecture series from The Great Courses, I decided to try U3A—The University of the Third Age—signing up for a programme of weekly presentations about the *100 Forests of the National Arboretum*. To join other elderly, lifelong learners with a love for trees, to improve my botanical knowledge of these wooded beings as there are several forest and park locations in and around Canberra, I frequently visit with superb specimens. Not being able to name or identify neighbourhood trees was a knowledge gap I wanted to fill with easy-paced tuition and digestible content.

With this year marking fifty years since I completed high school at Greytown in KwaZulu-Natal, South Africa, I decided to reactivate my Facebook account for the sole purpose of tracking down former classmates for an online reunion. I'd done something similar back in 2004 and since then had lost contact with most, keeping communication with only a few. It's been rewarding taking the lead to bring people, who share a unique bond, together again revitalising old friendships and beginning new ones. Scattered around the world, our geographical separation no barrier for the mix of modern communication systems to easily overcome, through WhatsApp, Messenger, FaceTime and Zoom.

In keeping with anniversary events, last year marked 25 years since Bobby, Louis and I arrived in Australia, to begin a new life, settling first in Wagga Wagga as newly minted migrants. To commemorate our arrival, I initiated two events, the first—late last year—a homely celebratory tea party with long standing local friends, and another—earlier this year—to deliver a speech to the Wagga Wagga District and Historical Society, about our migration journey and experience of living in the Riverina. As the inaugural Manager of the Museum of the Riverina, I had a close working relationship with the Historical Society at the time.

Given that there were several months when I was physically weak, emotionally tender and uncertain about my capabilities, these low-key social activities continued to build my confidence, confirming I hadn't lost my ability to organise, lead and perform in public, including delivering speeches. The events got me out of the house to solidify friendships and begin new ones. They also helped to replace the 'scared look in my eyes' I carried after my stroke—an observation made by a friend, many months later. In its place, I could wear a smile and present self-belief that despite the knock to my health and mobility, there was a life to live and milestones to celebrate.

For *spiritual growth*—another domain of post-traumatic growth—I turned to nature. To reconnect with nature as the place where I reenergise internally and find belonging—blending clarity of being and deeper meaning of life. A connection I'd lost before my stroke when caught in the busyness of daily routines and uncertainties about the future.

Six months after my medical emergency, I sought a therapeutic gardening course, having enjoyed and gained much from my veggie pod project, restoring strength and mobility to my weakened body and confidence to my mind that recovery was possible, patience being key. My online searches drew me to Nature Calling—to an alternative, eight-month ecotherapy course.

Since February, I've been eco-tuning, to reconnect, and deepen my connection with nature. Also, to enhance my awareness of nature's intrinsic power to bring healing to trauma, past and present, and provide renewed energy and purpose for life. A spiritual quest, to be soothed, inspired and guided by nature, for a *greater appreciation for life*, the fifth, and final, domain of post-traumatic growth.

DAY FOUR HUNDRED AND THIRTY-FIVE

Tuesday, 9th July 2024
50m indoor pool, Gungahlin Leisure Centre

Aqua Refresh

I have a lane to myself
dipping
into cool water
so soothing

I glide through the liquid
clean
clear, clarity of sight
so refreshing

Bubbles flow, waves ripple
settle
stilled by rubber rings
lines floating

Today's swim easy,
light
body and limbs in rhythmic flow
forward, propelling

In the beginning, post-stroke
a drunk frog
uncoordinated weak limbs
splashing in one spot

Now, smooth strokes again
speed
a revived stroke survivor
how good it feels

Body in motion, in water
buoyant
fluid emotions too
appreciation, floating free

Forwards, backwards lap after
lap
joyous children alongside
spirits rise, outside winter, inside summer fun.

DAY FOUR HUNDRED AND THIRTY-SEVEN

Thursday 11 July 2024
Chair, front garden, Bonner, ACT

Unmasked

Seated
bare feet, embedded in wet wood bark
mug of warm tea in hand

Still
morning mist, mark trees in silhouette
3 degrees, crispy chill

Breath
a steamy vapour trail
dissolving into frosted light

Birds
suspend flight, to welcome me
perched atop bare trees, steel lampposts

Signalling
to kin, and then to wing, to fly up high
squawks, screeches, melting into mistiness

Distinct
how lush, full leafed, and blooming
stands the protea, in mid-winter dress

Naked
the bare ash and flower-less gaura
a sheltered rose unseasonally in bloom

Cold
penetrates skin, an ice bath for muscles
refreshing, revitalising, restorative

Spirit
emerges, embodied alignment, headspace settled
I'm alive, protected by nature's grace.

DAY FOUR HUNDRED AND FORTY

Sunday, 14 July 2024
Royal Canberra Golf Club

Westbourne Woods

Between fairways we walk
admiring the trees
Driving, chipping, putting
left to others
Striding forth, behind motorised buggies
wheeled robots, racing across the turf.

Tradition, extending 43 years
second Sunday morning of each month
Friends of ACT Trees
retired foresters, botanists, arboriculturists
Lead tree-lovers through Westbourne Woods
alongside Lake Burley Griffin.

Inspired and planted by Charles Weston
horticulturist, officer-in-charge afforestation
Master experimenter with seeds
to forest treeless plains
Beautifying, greening, adding seasonal colour
to Canberra, when birthed a century plus ago.

Surprises rise in the morning sunlight
lone Mexican weeping pine
Dwarfed by the Monterey cypress
cluster of Bunya pine
Solitary, noble Sequoia
giant sentinel, watching over first green.

River Peppermint gum, green-domed centrepiece
Among Aleppo pines,
Through fallen rustic leaves of Pin oaks,
To Himalayan cypress in yellow flower
Alligator juniper
Species from around the world
Mature specimens helping to maintain our pristine air
Adding beauty, tranquility, to the bush capital.

DAY FOUR HUNDRED AND FORTY-SIX

Saturday, 20 July 2024
Home, Bonner, ACT

Haiku Moment

Bare feet in wood bark
skin-kissed by emerging sunlight
awareness . . . awakens within

DAY FOUR HUNDRED AND FORTY-EIGHT

Monday, 22 July 2024
Lindsay Pryor Arboretum, Canberra, ACT

Every circle has a centre

A special connection
paired cork oaks
planted the year I was born

My life rings mirrored
in tree limbs
mature, enduring, standing strong

I sit beneath, within, their canopy
enveloped, protected by green
taking counsel from living peers

Fire, storm, drought, wind, pests, urban encroachment
sum of experiences past, matching
maternal separation, adoption, hijacking, asbestos home, threatening stroke

Shared wounds, scars, regrowth and restorative living
I collect leaves from four directions
acorns from Mother Earth

Give thanks, to Great Spirit, in sky
absorb vital energy, tummy braced to bark
The past is passed, I shed old skin

Under the oaks, I look forward towards the future
to spring, next full moon on the horizon in Arcoora
Every circle has a centre, I'm getting close to finding mine.

DAY FOUR HUNDRED AND FIFTY-ONE

Thursday, 25 July 2024
Walk to Golden Sun Moth Hill with Bibi

West Wind

Up the ridge
thrust by westerly wind
rising east
to Sun Moth lookout

Sunlight casts shadows
beneath leaved limbs
My eyes turn south to
Brindabellas on far horizon

Refreshing stop
I salute the northern sun
head back west
Bibi and I alert

The past swept away
on cleansing gusts of nature's breath
Fresh vision, new purpose
emerging in its wake.

ONE YEAR, THREE MONTHS

Friday, 2 August 2024
Home, Bonner, ACT

Remembering Bojangles

Today is the first anniversary of farewelling Bojangles. Our friendship, feline to family, filled with joyful companionship, lasted 16 years.

The day it ended is still an unsettling memory.

After a session of carpet exercises, I stopped to make a mid-morning cup of tea. Through the kitchen window, I saw Bo outside in the garden, struggling to relieve himself. His back arched and contorted, stomach muscles taut, straining without success.

I watched as he ate some grass, which he sometimes did, causing him to vomit lightly, to release hair balls gathered in his throat from daily grooming. This time he struggled to spew, his frame remaining tense. Given his distress, I decided to take him to the vet.

With Bobby not home—as she'd returned to city-based office working—I believed I could drive to the nearest vet, 2 kms down the road, at the Amaroo shopping centre.

My concern for Bo overrode my hesitancy, as I hadn't driven my ute since being struck by stroke, three months before. My GP had only cleared me to drive a few days before, after passing an intensive medical examination. In the interim, I'd done a few short neighbourhood drives in the VW Golf.

Collecting Bo, I put him in his pet carrier, placing it on the front passenger seat, and drove down the road. I was tense and alert, concerned with his plight, while adjusting to the rhythms of my ute.

When we arrived, a sign on the front door, was not one I wanted to see: CLOSED.

Aware of another vet a kilometre down the road, I carried Bo back to the ute to make the journey. OPEN.

Bo and I waited patiently at reception while the receptionist finished a long telephone call. After explaining Bo's symptoms, her response, 'Are you an existing client?' Responding in the negative, 'Well, we can't see you then, the vet is busy and fully booked'.

My offer to wait for when the vet was available brought no change. The vet couldn't see us. Annoyed at the lack of concern and service, given Bo's distress, I carried Bo back to the ute.

Worried about him and driving longer distances after a long absence behind a wheel, I contemplated returning home and phoning Bobby to come and assist us. I decided to do neither, driving to Gungahlin instead, a few kilometres further down the road, where I knew of a third veterinary practice.

It too was closed!

One option remained, driving 14kms south to Brudine Veterinary Services, our former long-term family vet in Flynn, where we lived almost a decade before. They'd known Bo since he was a kitten.

Along the way I pulled over to give Bobby a call about Bo's situation and my movements.

Fourth time lucky! Bojangles and I found ourselves in familiar surroundings, seen by Dr Fiona, known to both of us, who was warm and welcoming even though we hadn't seen each other for a number of years.

After examining Bo, she took a series of blood tests. The diagnosis—not good. His white blood cell count was vitally low indicating his immune system was struggling to fight an infection. He was really sick, something he'd probably masked for some time. In hindsight, he hadn't been his usual self over the past month.

To my dismay, she recommended putting him to sleep. A verdict I wouldn't have accepted from any other vet. Dr Fiona knew Bo, his history, his age and the blood tests provided conclusive evidence of how ill he was. I trusted her judgement but disliked her recommendation—in its own right, and coming off a stressful morning.

First up, discovering his distress, driving my ute for the first time post-stroke, visiting four vets before we could be seen, and now this . . . Bo terminally ill and needing to be put down.

I was devastated.

Bojangles, who'd been a family member for 16 years, a rescued RSPCA kitten. Friend and companion who constantly shadowed me, in and outside the house.

The inspiration for Mr Petman, my former small business, building cat enclosures. The first of 400+ cat enclosures I built, was for him, to give him a safe outdoor, natural space when we moved into our Bonner home, to comply with local laws for protecting native wildlife.

Soft, cuddly, purring, communicative Bojangles. Desk companion when studying or writing. Warm leg cushion when watching TV. Playmate for indoor hide and seek. Bo who slept on my bed each night and who I fed each morning at 5.00am. His morning routine so precise, when clocks were reset twice a year for Daylight Saving, it took him about a week to reset his internal circadian rhythm.

He knew, as animals do, his time had come.

When I put him back into his carrier bag, he curled into a ball to sleep, showing no more interest in me or his surroundings—behaviour quite unlike him.

When Bobby arrived, the four of us retreated to a private, back room, to sit on a comfortable couch and witness Dr Fiona administer two injections.

My hand on his side, Bojangles life paused, and expired, gently. Peacefully, he drifted from this world at 2.20pm on 2 August 2023.

Five months to the day, after Dora—my mother—had passed away, and three months to the day, after I'd being struck by stroke. Of the three events, his passing, emotionally the hardest blow, indicating how much he meant to me.

Returning home with an empty carrier bag wasn't the outcome I'd had in my mind when I'd set out four hours earlier.

This latest misfortune a punctuation mark to a testing, traumatic and tragic six months.

A few weeks later, we collected Bo's ashes from the vet. Encased in a small wooden box, his name Mr Bojangles engraved on the lid, I placed the casket atop a bookcase in the master bedroom for ongoing visibility and presence.

Whether to grieve, or just to hold Bojangles' memory close, the space has become a slow-grow ceremonial zone to remember his life—as close friend and loyal companion who was constantly present, and a delight.

The ceremonial space incorporates several elements, in addition to his ashes. Petals that have fallen from single roses, from my garden, I regularly placed in a vase alongside; seashells, leaves, acorns and cones, I collected from significant trees or beaches from past travels. A variety of handcrafted objects—a modified copper pot, home-made candles cast from a cat head mould, a lamp made from fabric, created communally by Bobby, on one of her art retreats, all nesting beneath a framed print of a favourite mountain landscape.

Importantly, Bo's spirit is present offering nourishing memories, reflecting a cherished relationship that brought happiness to our household and enriched my life.

ONE YEAR, FOUR MONTHS

Monday 2 September 2024
Home, Bonner, ACT

Refreshed and Energised by Nature

Since February this year, I've been engaged in an Advanced Ecotherapy Course, delivered by Dr Geoff Berry of Nature Calling, ably co-presented by ecotherapist Charlotte Brown.

The bi-monthly, online course sessions, culminated in a five-day, in-person, nature retreat at a former Buddhist Centre in northern NSW.

I've just returned from this getaway, rejuvenated in mind, body and spirit.

Over the past seven months, I've purposely set out to reconnect with nature. To find deeper sense of being and belonging, coupling my sense of self to the natural world around me. To feel at home with myself and on this earth. My poetry reflects this quest, capturing moments spent with nature.

Along with ongoing exercise to restore my mobility, I've adopted practices to reestablish, and expand, the close affinity I've always felt with nature, but never allowed these leanings full expression.

The retreat was a significant continuation of my post-stroke recovery—physically, spiritually, mentally and relationally—complementing physiotherapy to include somatic and spiritual practices to create a package of holistic healing to enhance my wellness and wellbeing.

I purposely chose a 2,600km solo, return road trip in my ute from Canberra to Arcoora—the retreat venue. Given my limitations with physical stamina—compared to my pre-stroke capacity—I planned the road trip in stages, navigating smaller, inland roads, and avoiding major highways, motelling and camping along the way.

The intention was to boost my confidence as much as my physical endurance.

I eagerly embraced the 13-day challenge of long-distance driving, basic accommodation and frequent sight-seeing stops. The freedom of exploring country, on the open road, a pleasant adventure accompanying the main event—one of 19 participants who came to live, breathe, walk and sit within the protective canopy of ancient rainforest, to share learnings, and absorb nature's life-affirming power.

For some readers, this might appear a personal indulgence into woo-woo-land. A sign that I'd lost my marbles, with a juvenile urge to return to 1970s hippie culture, spaced out in drug-filled stupor, exhilarated by free range sex and a Woodstock soundtrack! How far off the mark you'd be.

Let's sit quietly for a moment in grounded space.

Ecopsychology is an established discipline of enquiry and ecotherapy, as applied practice, explores and recognises the ecological relation of living things to their environment. A key tenet is that human beings are part of a larger ecological system—the broader world of living things—the natural world, or what we often refer to, as nature.

Psychology itself holds interest in the human psyche—the study of mind. For many earlier scholars and earth's people, understanding soul, rather than mind, was the core interest. That part of human nature sitting above, outside and beyond mental cognition that we connect to, or attune with, through creative and relational bonds between ourselves and nature. An awareness of our human artistry, intuition and spirituality that allows us to rest in the stillness of being or to experience qualities of the divine. The latter often experienced in nature—especially for indigenous peoples worldwide.

Globally and cross culturally, there is widespread and growing recognition that human beings are intimately connected with their natural world and that human, industrial and consumer-driven enterprise—recent past and daily present—places enormous pressure on the sustainable functioning of the natural world, our world. A pressure that is detrimental to human health, individually and collectively, and to the earth, our home that protects, feeds and nurtures all living creatures.

This recognises that our shared, natural living world holds inter-and co-dependency for essential wellness of being. That in appreciating and enjoying what nature offers, we not only recognise its intrinsic life force and holistic healing properties, but more—step up to respect and protect them. To be advocates for the precious health-wealth nature holds for sustaining all life.

Given that this book is about my post-stroke recovery, now isn't the time to digress into advancing the philosophy underpinning ecopsychology and its practical expression, ecotherapy. Nonetheless, I do encourage those who wish to explore this field to read the pioneer thinkers and practitioners who laid the groundwork for many to follow, notably the deep ecology concepts articulated by Norwegian philosopher, Arne Naess, Theodore Roszak's seminal work, *The Voice of the Earth: An Exploration of Ecopsychology* and Harold Clinebell's, *Ecotherapy: Healing ourselves, healing the earth.*

These thinkers have all sown the seeds for propagating the re-awareness of respecting, and being open, to nature's intelligence, recognised in many cultural traditions, as reliable ancient wisdom and guidance. The goal, to reconnect with the natural world to heal the human psyche and the earth, using knowledge that can sit beside, and work in parallel, with contemporary technological innovation, to sustain a liveable world for all.

Other significant works include *Spiritual Ecology: The Cry of the Earth*, edited by Llewellyn Vaughan-Lee; any writings by Joanna Macy, especially *Coming Back to Life: The Updated Guide to the Work that Reconnects*, co-authored with Molly Brown; John Swanson's, *Communing with Nature: A guidebook for enhancing your relationship with the living earth*; and lastly, our course book, *Ecotherapy: healing with nature in mind*, edited by Linda Buzzell and Craig Chalquist.

The titles of these compilations succinctly capture the context and intention of nature therapy—a recognition of, and respect for, the natural world and an invitation to reconnect with nature, individually and collectively, to open ourselves to its presence as a living container for holistic good health. In communing with nature, our physical, mental, spiritual and relational domains become connected to a deeper life force, improving wellness and wellbeing, bring meaning to existence and providing better life satisfaction.

My own affinity with nature—as primary place of inspiration, reflection, comfort and play—was born and nurtured during childhood when the outdoors—the front and backyards of our suburban home—provided a safe, pleasurable haven in which to explore and rest. I learnt early to appreciate fresh air, sunlight, trees, plants and animals as our household pets included dogs, cats, canaries, bantams and chickens.

Being an adopted child, I experienced a sensory lapse of deep belonging with family, as my original biological ties were taken from me when assigned a new identity and family at birth. I was fortunate to receive a loving and kind replacement family, though in depth of primary and sensory connection, they remained foreign, requiring a complex adaptation when I set out to begin life.

Living with a fractured identity without the grounding of biological kin, my immediate interactions with the world were tethered to feelings of bewilderment, uncertainty and vigilance.

As a consequence, an inner tension evolved within me leading to a confusing headspace characterised by not knowing who I was and relationally, where I fitted in the world. As a newborn without mother, I was cast into liminality, suspended in the middle of the air, scarred by a deep sense of abandonment.

Being in, and with, nature became a refuge. Being active outdoors dissolved any feelings of loneliness, providing me with a comfort that I belonged somewhere. I developed a quiet knowing—in head, heart and spirit—that in nature there was a mysterious sense of connection, absent in family life. By contrast, in the family home I felt, at worst, like an intruder, at best, a guest. Often a stranger to myself and those around me. Nature became a friend, a place for playful activity and safe belonging. This sense of being I held tightly, silently and privately as it was too important to lose or have taken from me.

My nature connection expanded in my adolescent years when I was fortunate to have annual seaside holidays at caravan parks or at a relative's coastal farm. These experiences widened my external world and introduced me to superb land- and seascapes, to African wildlife and domestic farm animals, creating an appreciation for the natural world and living creatures.

Ever since, as I've navigated through life stages, successfully, or to stumble and fall before picking myself up again, the pull of green or blue natural spaces has remained strong. Regularly I found myself drawn to forests, mountains, savannah or the oceans, lakes and rivers to rest, replenish depleted energy or stabilise the comfortable felt sense of being home.

This deep sensory presence of nature frequently influenced my choices of where I wanted to live and work—to set up a home base. Often, I'd choose locations of exquisite natural beauty, Cape Town for example, or seasonal, garden cities, with abundant green space, low population density, absence of polluting industries and ease of access to natural bushland—with Canberra a fine exemplar.

To this day, whenever I've being fortunate to travel, especially to large cities around the world—Sydney, Tokyo, London and Hamburg come to mind—upon arrival in these metropolises, it wouldn't take long before I'd be drawn to their parks, gardens, lakes and waterways, as this is where I felt most comfortable.

My nature connection, though recognised early in life, remained a backdrop, rather than a centrepiece, as I directed primary energy to daily life performance—work, study and family as focus points while continually juggling—mentally and emotionally—a strong desire to know my ancestry, to fill the hole in my being with belonging. To exchange being a 'something' with a fractured identity, to 'someone' with clear familial and grounded connections. As a recipient of a closed adoption order, it was decades before I could search and have hope of reconnecting with biological kin. Within my personal world, nature stepped in to become my surrogate family, bestowing a sense of true belonging.

I'm thankful for my early childhood nature experiences as the personal memories I hold, of a safe haven, is the place I return when in crisis, not least when struck by the stroke last year.

Six months post-stroke, when the shock of what had hit me settled, and through an extensive period of physiotherapy—recounted in earlier narrative—allowed me to regain my functional mobility, notwithstanding being weaker and wobbly on my feet. I looked for ways to strengthen and expand my nature connection, beginning with sitting, walking and gardening outdoors. The presence of nature such a valuable ally in my recovery, the stroke forced me to take the relationship to another level.

In November 2023, I looked up therapeutic gardening courses online. When none appealed, I expanded my Google searches leading me to Nature Calling, and the advanced ecotherapy course I enrolled in and will soon complete.

For the past seven months, I've placed my being in the presence of nature, observing, noticing and listening to Mother Earth, what she can teach me. To become more aware and connected to my 'ecological self', the term first used by Arnold Naess. The acknowledgement that as a human being I'm not separate from, nor superior to, nature. For my fellow human beings, and I, to continue to flourish on this earth, we need to respect and appreciate the complex natural ecosystems within our world. To value, not overuse them as an open warehouse for unsustainable exploitation or consumption, targeted at material wealth alone. Crucially, we have the intellectual and technological smarts to recognise nature's intrinsic life sustaining value, as a prerequisite for quality of life and good health for all, everywhere.

My ideal for sustainable holistic health begins at home, in my front garden, sit spotting. This is a traditional practice of finding a comfortable place to sit quietly with, and in, nature. And while seated, tune into my senses and my immediate surroundings, consciously communing with nature, as a powerful grounding practice.

Recommended as a daily, or regular practice, in the one spot I sit in a chair in my front garden, avoiding any need to drive or walk to my chosen nature spot. The terraced garden providing some privacy, while offering uninterrupted views up and down the tree-lined street. A convenient and practical choice, as most of my sessions occur at sunrise.

Over many mornings, I've witnessed the unfolding seasons, my bare feet embedded in the wood bark of my roses, while enjoying the day's first cup of tea. Occasionally, I'd have a repeat session later in the day or at night.

The simplicity of sitting quietly, attentively observing nature, without other distractions, empowers sensory awareness. To see, smell, hear, taste, touch and holistically feel, grounding self to nature. Enriching the experience of being alive in the fullness of body, mind and spirit.

Along with frequency of practice, it's important I not self-distract—I leave my mobile phone, any reading or writing materials, inside the house so I can remain fully present in nature for 15 - 20 minutes, sometimes longer.

Importantly, the benefits come from practice, not from description.

Go out into nature, find your comfortable sit spot, tune into your senses, and be open for a gradual transformation of being. Practice, regularly—daily if you can—to experience the rewards of practice. Bring intent as if learning to play a musical instrument or speak a new language.

Sit spotting along with guided meditation—which I've practiced regularly for over a year now—together with nature walking and forest bathing—which I've referenced in earlier pages or through my poetry—have accumulated, much like compound interest, to stimulate my wellness and improve my wellbeing. Collectively, they've facilitated a steady, ongoing post-stroke recovery, once formal physiotherapy ended. Vital to my health and wellbeing, the practices align to the stroke survivor mantra—*there is no end date to recovery*.

By the time I'd arrived at Arcoora to join the other retreat participants, we'd engaged in thirteen online group sessions, exploring how to welcome ourselves back to nature and to self. To rebalance our beings, especially when having suffered any of life's menu of traumas, whether physically, mentally, emotionally, or having lost connection relationally, or with our spirituality. To ground our being, back to nature. To recognise that nature's intelligence has a voice worth listening to.

As a group we'd come together to begin to understand and feel what we could do and be, to process feelings, harms and hurts. Of loss, separation, grief and deep emotional pain, caused by violations—physical or emotional abuse, childhood trauma, parental challenges, physical illness, work stress, burnout or as witnesses to the destruction of our living planet. Complex and layered trauma that disorientates, often spirals out of control, leaving feelings of hopelessness and helplessness.

In between our two-hour, fortnightly, online sessions we'd dug deep into set readings, practical exercises and themes for group conversations, as well as being encouraged to journal our experience and complete a monthly assignment. The latter a written essay, artwork, photograph, poem or a journal entry, acknowledging that people learn and express their learnings and insights in different ways, especially when we open ourselves to all our senses, requiring flexible mediums for expression.

Given our earlier online interactions, a level of mutual trust and support had been established, allowing us to expand our learning experience, tuning into nature *in situ*, individually and collectively.

I arrived at Arcoora with an open mind and heart, coupled with strong intent, to fully participate in all the activities. Undeterred, I was the oldest member present and one of only three males. For the first time in my life, I accepted a self-perception of elder, drawing upon, and sharing, the depths of my life experience, while listening to the stories of others.

Encouraged to express our full sensory experience through meditation, communal ceremony, creative art practices, physical movement, individual contemplation exercises and encircled group reflection, I gave practical expression to these activities, reassured of being held in a safe space, by nature and one another. My heartfelt intent to be whole in myself, so that I could be of service to others.

Importantly, we practiced the art of deep listening—listening to ourselves, others and nature in respectful silence—absorbing, holding, deep emotion whenever uncomfortable or affirming feelings, arose.

And often they did. Deep-rooted emotion from previous loss, separation, grief or violation leading to fear, anger, or feelings of sadness, despair or rejection.

As the days unfolded, immersed in restorative practices within nature, shifts began to appear, observable to ourselves and to each other. Some more noticeable than others, as internal trauma processing—to settle within, gain new direction or life purpose—incubates at its own pace—it's neither competitive, nor predictable. Insights and embodied renewal often arise unexpectedly, in the moment or later in the course of daily living.

It was humbling to witness shifts of surprise, joy, clarity, compassion, love or renewed hope when they emerged within our psyches. Somatically, our bodies releasing tension, and a gamut of emotions, to settle into moments of harmonious being. Clarity of choice, a relaxed body, inspired inner spirit—communally shared—ebbing and flowing throughout each day.

Forty years ago, Arcoora was built by monks to create a Buddhist centre, their residency lasting three decades. The centrepiece, a wooden and glass, square-shaped temple or 'gompa', on a hilltop amongst mature trees. The large, modest and unembellished hall still holds a soothing, spiritual presence. When sitting, cross-legged on cushions on the wooden patina floor, the building appears to float, suspended among tree trunks, resembling a giant tree house. Ideal for reconnecting with nature and the spiritual realm.

Each morning, we began the day in this sacred assembly space with NIA (Neuromuscular Integrative Action). A gentle impact exercise incorporating movements from dance, martial arts and yoga—among other sharings. A body-centred awareness practice, NIA aims to improve physical flexibility, agility, mobility, stability, strength and co-ordination. Exercise is meant to be joyous and uplifting, giving your body free licence to move comfortably, in its own way.

I was unfamiliar with NIA prior to the retreat and instantly took to the practice. I particularly enjoyed the exercise of retracing my body's first five stages of development, moving from embryonic to creeping, crawling, standing and walking. As a stroke survivor needing to retrain my brain to regain finer motor skills, NIA provided a whole new set of fit-for-purpose, stimulating exercises.

Guided meditation followed NIA, our bodies, minds and spirits offered the opportunity to embrace stillness and sense life force, before breakfast. To set ourselves up for the day's activities equipped with courage and intent. One of my most enduring memories of the retreat is sitting in a treescape of green, touched by the emerging sunlight, filtering through the windows, embraced by heart sense and the collective calmness of others, seated in deep meditation.

I've visited cathedrals and churches all over the world—including iconic Christian sites in Nazareth, Bethlehem and Jerusalem. I've participated in the ceremony of mass hundreds of times in my early life, yet none of these visits or experiences matches the sense of spiritual presence I felt within, when entering the Arcoora sacred assembly space for a solitary vigil, or when seated in a circle, meditating or in communal ceremony, listening to others.

Daily, after breakfast, we'd return to the assembly space for a sensory check-in and outline of the day's activities. On the first day, a walk into the forest, to become familiar with the landscape, identify a personal sit spot or future pathway, in preparation for paired sessions. The latter, to buddy up, one as counsellor, the second as client, walking out into the living, natural landscape, to combine therapeutic intention with nature's inherent ability to heal. Multiple dyad conversations occurred, with each of us given more than one opportunity to be a counsellor or client. After each session, an intensive feedback discussion followed, counsellors in one pod, clients in another.

Earlier, to solidify connection, remembrance or as a messenger, we collected a single object from nature, bearing personal significance or attraction. A guiding symbol, blessed by nature, we believed worthy of being placed on a wooden table at the front of the assembly space. All our individual objects left there until the final morning, before returning them to nature.

I was drawn to the bright orange, white and blue petals of a strelitzia flower, its distinctive birdlike shape atop a smooth long stem. Known as the 'Bird of Paradise', several flowering plants were present close to the entrance of the assembly space.

Extended an invitation to create a visual expression of our life, as a river, we collected paint, pastels, pen and paper to illustrate our journey, and on a separate day, got our hands messy embedding them in raw clay, for a more tactile experience, shaping an animal or natural object, as a symbol of who we were or had become.

Seated on the floor, we completed both exercises in pairs or in solitary engagement. After the river painting exercise, our compositions and their symbolism were discussed, before laying them out on the floor, in front of the ceremonial altar space. In doing so, natural lines, shapes and colours, naturally began to emerge, to link them all together in continuous flow. Spellbound, we stood back, seeing our colourful creations, as if by some mysterious design, become one artwork—a composite mosaic of life experience, bestowed with belonging.

My clay work produced a stylised tree and two ringed faces—the first, my startled stroke face, the other a smiling face, representative of my current state of being.

One morning, we gathered in the sacred assembly space for an hour-long, communal grief circle ceremony. To voluntarily share and release, in a secure, safe space, troubling states of being, characterised by deep feelings of anger, sadness, grief or loss, to be witnessed by others in respectful and attentive silence. Whatever the emotional pain expressed in the circle, once released, was validated by the witnesses through a single verbal affirmation. The exercise, both a release and expression of bare honesty and inner truth telling—intense, confronting, profoundly emotionally and spiritually healing.

Under clear skies and a near full moon, we gathered in the darkened assembly space to choose an animal spirit and enact, through creative movement, the animal's motion or behaviour traits.

Embracing this animal spirit, as totemic guide, to further deepen our nature connection. To rebalance being and realign direction for bringing clarity of purpose to our lives.

Within my psyche, the image of a lion spontaneously appeared. A surprise, as my normal cognitive ignition would have chosen either an elephant or a cow, as both animals have held symbolic significance for me in past. And cows still do.

Embodying the movement of a lion across the floor, I pondered the connection, why a lion? Lions are strong, independent, self-sufficient, leaders. Figuratively, lion traits embody power, intention and growth, the energies I'd brought to the retreat and previously set for my post-stroke recovery. In addition, lions express anger and aggression when challenged or cornered, behaviours not always effective for bringing about change without harm. Particularly, self-directed harm. While moving on all fours across the floor, an awareness emerged of giving myself greater agency, to be more assertive and employ strategies of persuasion, negotiation and diplomacy, as tools for calmer living.

Staying in totemic mindset, I recognised, since struck by the stroke, I'd sought qualities of strength and resilience to regain strength and clarity—physically, emotionally and spiritually.

In tandem with mindful intent, I allowed myself to be emotionally vulnerable and expose feelings of sadness, hurt and grief—long suppressed. To let them rise and to release them. When speaking in session, I'd often choke with emotion, prompting a spontaneous beating of my heart with my hand, to dislodge the embodied blockage.

The appearance of a lion as guiding totem implanted my life journey with a layer of nature-given-guidance, and a discussion point, as after the activity, group members discussed their own totem animal, while seated around a glowing log fire under full moonlight. To make shifts towards wholesome personal growth, for greater awareness.

In my case, the realisation that anger, impatience and perfectionism undermine healthy wellbeing.

One evening, I returned to the assembly space to deliver a poetry writing workshop to six of my fellow participants, guiding them through a sequence of creative exercises to craft their own poem about a significant life experience.

Beginning with a calming jazz soundtrack, the musical interlude providing a transition space to step out of supper mode and into writing mode. Before we started, I gifted each person with a pen and personal notebook, the latter, handmade weeks before by Bobby.

The opening act, a fun activity to write and share a six-word autobiography in ten minutes.

To complete the longer composition, a further 20 to 25 minutes quickly passed. Once done we shared our crafted words, reciting them in our own voices, to be heard, and importantly, listened to, without censure or analysis. Being open-hearted, to value the sharing as an intimate and vulnerable expression of being.

Poetry, as a form of expressive writing, does open creative channels to our emotional and spiritual centres, offering personal healing and growth, similar to the embodied benefits received from art, meditation, sit spotting, prayer or journaling practices.

As an introvert, poetry helps me, as a sensory being, to integrate thought, with deep feelings and spiritual connection, to express fullness of being in written form. To grasp, and share, key experiences as they unfold as pivotal moments of insight, held with joy, sadness or other emotion. For millennia, people have embraced creative expression, in all forms, poetry being one in the pool of music, dance, theatre, painting, singing, storytelling and writing that enliven and enrich the performing, visual and literary arts that are open to all.

To this list we could add architectural nature design, as we were divided into two groups to create a spirit house outside, in the vicinity, of the assembly space, using natural or other materials we could find without damaging the environment. Once built, each group invited the other to visit their spirit house—to be welcomed in ritual ceremony, of our making. Presented as a competitive exercise, it needn't have been, as both parties managed to harness the energy of team dynamics collaboratively, to create a pair of spirit houses, grounded in nature, along with ceremonies of welcome, that included singing, body painting and placement of gifts, as spiritual offerings. Doing so under grey skies and light drizzle added further mystery, as joyful delight flowed through both ceremonies.

Before dawn, on the final morning, I returned to the assembly space to sit in quiet soltitude, reflecting on the richness and depth of my sensory experience. Of placing myself, together with others, in therapeutic space with nature, actively creating life skills and new pathways for creating and sustaining better wellness. In the stillness of spirit and presence of nature, I wrote:

In retreat
beginning anew
I prepare
to advance
into the future.

I've spoken
personal stories
of loss
sadness
deep grief
received insight.

I've being listened to
heard by others
with open hearts

attentive minds
welcoming spirits.

My exposed wounds
dressed by collective caring
of kindred souls
open
to nature healing.

My fragile, inner nature
held, honoured
in safeness
tended by respectful listening
wrapped by warm hugs
encouraging conversation
silence when needed.

My knowing
body sensing
spiritual depths
enlightened by fresh insight
nourishing physical restoration
touched by nature's inspiration

On the cusp of transition
to step out
and explore new pathways
I depart strengthened
by nature, human kindness
and generosity
abundant in this sacred space
among the rain forest.

Later that morning, in the final activity, we collected our natural object from the ceremonial altar, along with our crafted clay objects, to place them outside at a spot of our choosing. When lifting the two circular faces representing my stroke-self and post-stroke-self, the former crumbled in my hands, while the latter remained intact.

Returning to the spirit house I'd helped build, I scattered the pieces of stroke-self on the ground and lifting the smiling clay face of my current self, I placed it on the altar, between the trunks, amidst the Camellia flowers, to nestle beside all the other offerings.

Like my fellow participants, I'd come to Arcoora to awaken the restorative power of nature within me to progress my post-stroke healing, and to release layers of trapped emotional energy that had lain dormant for years. I'd come to refresh my mind, rejuvenate my body and open my spirit. Five days in, I was satisfied, to venture forth, and continue my life journey.

DAY . . .

2 October 2024

Home, Bonner, ACT

The future

On the eve of the spring equinox, I attended a communal grief circle at Wamboin, NSW. Joining a group of fifteen people, none who I knew or had met before. Sitting on the lawn, in front of a private residence, the north-westerly wind blew strong and cold throughout the four-hour ceremony. It took courage and commitment from all attendees to stay present and face whatever left them unsettled within.

A week before, the ecotherapy course had ended with the final post retreat online session. With the conclusion of the course and shifting seasons, I felt the need to attend the grief circle as a transition point to bring this phase of my recovery to a close.

I'm fortunate my life continues in wholesome fullness post-stroke. The last eighteen months of my life—reflected in the pages of this book—have had their measure of challenge and difficulty, not least a sequence of personal losses that shook my core.

Spinning me into an orbit of unknowns: what to do, and be, in retirement after ceasing formal work; losing Dora—my mother, Bojangles—my pet cat, and my former able-bodied self; having to regain my mobility.

These life-turning events are valid invitations to grieve. To acknowledge and accept them as well as release any emotional pain or mental confusion that accompanied each loss. And to find connection to propel me forward, gathering life-affirming energy that sits in nature, lies within me, or gifted by the generosity and kindness of others. From close family or friends—old and new— along with pets, garden plants at home, the beauty of wider nature.

These recent events have compelled me to adapt, to sink or to swim, but to what shoreline?

During the grief circle, I wrote a short poem, which I polished a day later at home. Its insights succinctly cover my journey over the past year-and-a-half with a fragile quality to take into the future.

Hope

The wind blows
strongly

Icy blasts
of late winter chill

Sweeping away
the anguish and hurt

Recent losses
lingering grief

Dora, mother
old Thomas, pre-stroke self

Bojangles, feline friend
the natural world, under threat

*Seasonal change
brings transition*

*The equinox, spring, signals
new beginnings*

*Hope for lighter
fresher, gentler breeze*

*Sunshine, nourishing warmth
stillness, less icy wind.*

The practice of ceremony in, and with, nature, sometimes with physical discomfort, though without threat, is viscerally charged. Tapping into felt experience, emotionally, and deeper still, sensing the spiritual quality, in the moment, is energising. Expressing sensory engagement with ourselves in nature and in communion with others, as a combination, heightens awareness of being.

Our energy shifts within, we become open, sensitive beyond description—across all our sensory domains—even when we try to capture the encounter in words. We feel, deep within, messaging that is personal, private, parabolic. We momentarily suspend reason, judgment, and the need to measure.

In ceremony, performed collectively, a sense of oneness emerges, an affirming life sense, charged with emotion, joyful or subdued—and spiritual direction, clarity received or a call for more reflection. The messaging has a precious quality, prompting a mental urge to want to hold it indefinitely, to create a keepsake. For me, I craft words in flow, to mirror the life experience. Something for the mind to grasp when it inevitably returns, seeking understanding or wanting to explain, desiring to tell. There is no need, having lived the ceremony, felt the sensory awareness, that is enough. Best to sit with it, enact the symbolic messaging.

I will continue working on my physical recovery practicing a range of exercises blended from many different sources. To support my body and stimulate my brain to refine and strengthen the neural connections to enable finer motor skills to be stable on my feet and to maintain good health. My upper right limb strength and mobility is at 90%, my lower limbs at 85%.

The process a dual challenge: a naturally ageing body in need of stable and flexible mobility now, and to serve my ageing body in the future, when I enter my 70s, even my 80s.

Having reached my late 60s, my desire is for quality of life, rather than longevity of life. If the two happen to coincide, better the good fortune.

The life package I work towards, and hopefully will be surrounded by, has these attributes: good physical health, including able-bodied mobility—ideally without pain—along with mental clarity, coupled with emotional stability and spiritual depth, bolstered by relational connection with nature, drawing upon its nourishing vitality, and human friends who hold similar values, aspiring for contentment of being. Obviously, life doesn't come with guarantees, offer certainty, nor promise health or assure wealth. Nonetheless, these factors frame my future leanings, as they are worth striving for.

I intend to remain an active partner in my own physical recovery, bringing courage and determination, coupled with humility and appreciation. I'm grateful for what I have—in human qualities, friendships and nature. For the life I've led and for what is still to unfold.

THANK YOU

Nature, on earth, our natural home for all—from the very beginning. We have a collective obligation to protect, preserve and sustain our natural world. To ensure that we have a healthy life-sustaining home, for all living beings now, and into the future.

I would not be as well, nor as mobile as I am today, without the excellent early medical intervention and attention I received from neurologists, doctors, nurses, physiotherapists and occupational therapists at the former Calvary Hospital (now North Canberra Hospital) and at the University of Canberra Hospital Rehabilitation Centre. I'm perennially thankful for the medical treatment I received. A credit to the public health system.

Bobby, like many partners who assume roles as stand-in carers, had to carry additional responsibilities and the burden of uncertainty when I turned our stable life upside down. She stood up, when I fell down. I'm forever grateful for your unwavering equanimity and support through my ongoing rehabilitation.

Louis, for the support given to his mother, and to me, under stressful life circumstances, having to deal with parental illness while completing a Master's degree in psychology.

A special mention to good friend, Sandy Clugston, who completed the cat tunnel installation that I left unfinished at the client when struck by stroke, and for the regular catch-ups, whether for coffee/tea, short or longer walks, and garden service assistance, over the course of my recovery.

Bobby and I certainly appreciated the visits in hospital, and at home, in the aftermath of my stroke. We sincerely thank the following friends for giving of their time and showing compassion: Catherine Lynch; Sandy Clugston and Kerry Blackburn; Rooney and Trish Galloway; Ann and Tim Leske; Glenda Smith; Michael Goss; Christine Draper, Peter Blackman; Sam Senaratne; Gemma Black and David Nuttal; Bridget and Peter Knaus; Di Seath; Valda Johnson; Betty Mills and Robbie Lawrence; Rodney Smith; Sue Allen; Lisa Teasdale; Lisa Beattie, Nathan, Kerrie-Anne and Arthur Nguyen; Sunny, Clarissa and Gwenth Lai; Jason, Grace, Ethan and Blake Guo and Graham Goosen.

In addition, Bobby acknowledges all the kind messages and support she received from many people during the first three weeks of personal upheaval, particularly from her network of art colleagues.

Similarly, I convey my heartfelt thanks to friends and family for their good wishes received online: Jo-Ann Sparrow, June Webber, David Bradley, Birgitt Horn, Val Griffiths, Derek Wrankmore, Nicole Porter, Kylie Carman-Brown, Anne Else, Maria Haenga-Collins, Charlotte Smith, Louise Doyle, Roslyn Russell, Esther Esmyol, Claudia Ceresa, Claire Barrow, Rosie Newbigging, Gail Lecce, Lynne Abrahamson, Carol Bishop, Inge Wolter-Grazek, Doris Reynolds, Roland Mastnak, Fritz Mastnak, Gary Coles, Sue Collier, Dorria Watt, Amber Land, Elizabeth Kelly, Martin Wells, Pam and Keith Warburton, Cathy and Don Galvin, Debbie and Noel Young, Monica and Rob Pease, Gereon Schnippenkoetter, Julie Armstrong, Christian Wolter and Bastian Wolter.

To Brian McArthur, former school buddy and friend, for proofreading the raw manuscript of this book and offering literary advice to improve my work. Much appreciated.

Geoff Berry, Charlotte Brown, Silvana Nossiter, Marion Miller and my co-participants who shared the ecotherapy course together—the experience, as well as the learnings received from you all were inspiring and restorative.

My former classmates at Greytown High School, who have participated this year in the 50th anniversary of finishing school together—it's been a pleasure to orchestrate our reunion online to revive memories of 1974 and create new ones.

In a similar vein, to members of the Waterfront Rotary Club in Cape Town, the continuing friendships over the past 32 years mean a lot to me, as is seeing my former club continue to flourish as a humanitarian service organisation.

GLOSSARY

ACT	Australian Capital Territory
Bibi	Fox terrier, our pet dog
Bobo	Bojangles, my late pet cat
CAT Scan	Computed Axial Tomography Scan
COVID	An acute disease in humans caused by a coronavirus that became a pandemic in 2020
COWs	Computer on Wheels
FB	Facebook
FES	Functional Electric Stimulation
Gompa	Buddhist temple or monastery
Koeksister	Afrikaans word for a sticky, crisp, sweet pastry
Lekker	Afrikaans word meaning 'nice' or 'very nice'
MRI	Magnetic Resonance Imaging
NIA	Neuromuscular Integrative Action
Mr Petman	Name of my former small business
OT	Occupational Therapist
PTG	Post Traumatic Growth
NSW	New South Wales
Samoosa	A fried pastry with savoury filling originating from Southeast Asia popular in South Africa
Statin	Medicine designed to lower levels of low-density lipoprotein (LDL) cholesterol in the blood

UC University of Canberra
WFH Work from home

RESOURCES CITED AND COURSES COMPLETED

(In chronological sequence as they appear in text)

- Stroke Foundation, *My Stroke Journey: A book for survivors of stroke, families and carers*
- Simone Dorsch, Brian Beh & Stephanie Ho, *The Brain that changes: Neuroplasticity and stroke rehabilitation* (one hour lecture at University of Canberra Hospital)
- Owen Bullock, *Poetry and Wellbeing Workshop* (University of Canberra Hospital)
- Norman Doidge, *The Brain That Changes Itself*
- Robert McCrum, *My Year Off—Recovering Life After a Stroke*
- Molly Birkholm, *Building Your Resilience: Finding Meaning in Adversity* (online course)
- Molly Birkholm, *iRest: Integrative Restoration Yoga Nidra for Deep Relaxation* (online course)
- Jason Satterfield, *Mind-Body Medicine: The New Science of Optimal Health* (online course)
- *Adopt Perspective*, podcast for people affected by adoption, produced by Jo-Ann Sparrow, for Jigsaw Queensland (episodes 1st and 15th November 2023)
- Harvard Health Publishing, *Managing Your Cholesterol* (online course)
- PubMed Central (PMC), Numerous online articles about statin medication and its side effects, sourced from the archive of

biomedical and life sciences journal literature at the U.S. National Institutes of Health's National Library of Medicine.
- Russ Harris, *The Reality Slap*
- Nature Calling, *Advanced Ecotherapy Course* (eight months duration, online and 5-day in person retreat)
- Jan Morgan, *Trees of the Arboretum* (University of Third Age in-person course)
- Theodore Roszak, *The Voice of the Earth: An Exploration of Ecopsychology*
- Harold Clinebell, *Ecotherapy: Healing ourselves, healing the earth*
- Llewellyn Vaughan-Lee (editor), *Spiritual Ecology: The Cry of the Earth*
- Joanna Macy & Molly Brown, *Coming Back to Life: The Updated Guide to the Work that Reconnects*
- John Swanson, *Communing with Nature: A guidebook for enhancing your relationship with the living earth*
- Linda Buzzell & Craig Chalquist, *Ecotherapy: healing with nature in mind*
- Mandi Byron, Ink & Insight Art Therapy & Counselling and Sam Hawker of Garden Kitchen Witch*n, *Grief Circle—Spring Equinox*

MEDICAL ALERT!

If you suspect a stroke, apply the **F.A.S.T** test:

Face —check the face for any facial droop.

Arms —is there an inability to lift arms?

Speech —is speech slurred?

Time—time is critical.

If the above signs are present call medical emergency at once.

www.ingramcontent.com/pod-product-compliance
Ingram Content Group Australia Pty Ltd
76 Discovery Rd, Dandenong South VIC 3175, AU
AUHW011256301224

404783AU00002B/2